THE COMPLETE DIVERTICULITIS COOKBOOK FOR BEGINNERS

1200 Days Of Clear Liquid, Low Residue And High Fiber Recipes To Soothe Digestive System | With 28-Day Meal Plan Following 3-Stage Nutrition Guide To Manage And Prevent Flare-Ups

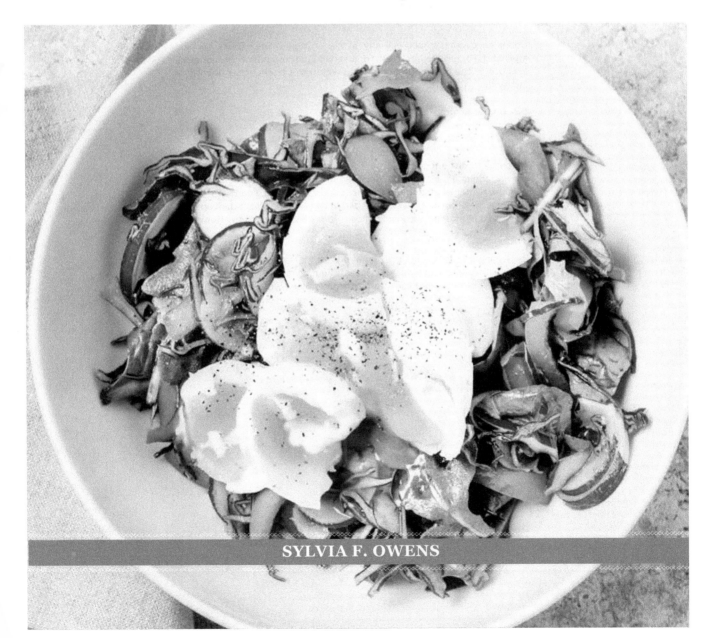

SYLVIA F. OWENS

Copyright© 2022 By Sylvia F. Owens Rights Reserved

This book is copyright protected. It is only for personal use. You cannot amend, distribute, sell, use, quote or paraphrase any part of the content within this book, without the consent of the author or publisher.

Under no circumstances will any blame or legal responsibility be held against the publisher, or author, for any damages, reparation, or monetary loss due to the information contained within this book, either directly or indirectly.

Disclaimer Notice:

Please note the information contained within this document is for educational and entertainment purposes only. All effort has been executed to present accurate, up to date, reliable, complete information. No warranties of any kind are declared or implied. Readers acknowledge that the author is not engaged in the rendering of legal, financial, medical or professional advice. The content within this book has been derived from various sources. Please consult a licensed professional before attempting any techniques outlined in this book.

By reading this document, the reader agrees that under no circumstances is the author responsible for any losses, direct or indirect, that are incurred as a result of the use of the information contained within this document, including, but not limited to, errors, omissions, or inaccuracies.

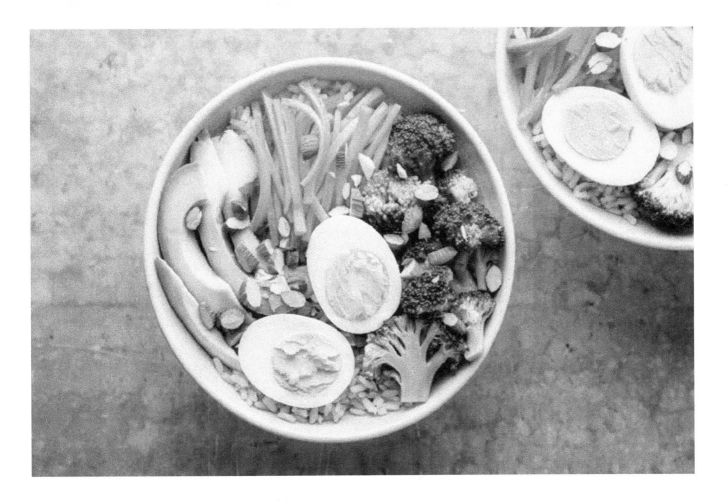

Table of Contents

Introduction	1
Chapter 1	
Understanding the Link Between Diverticulitis and Fiber	2
Risk Factors for Diverticulitis	3
Obesity	3
Red Meat Diet	3
Sedentary Lifestyle	4
Age	4
What Foods to Avoid	4
Seeds	4
Raw Veggies	4
Corn	4
Spicy Food	4
Cruciferous Vegetables	5
Dairy	5
Greasy Fast Food	5
Alcohol	5
Dealing with Diverticulitis Flare-Ups with Antibiotics	5
Using Probiotics to Manage Diverticulitis	5
Chapter 2	
Treatments and Care for Diverticulitis	6
Treating Uncomplicated Diverticulitis	7
Treating Complicated Diverticulitis	7
What to Expect After Surgery	9
How Do You Adhere to a Diet?	9

Chapter 3	
28-Day Meal Plans	11
Week 1	12
Week 2	12
Week 3	13
Week 4	13
Chapter 4	
Breakfast Recipes	14
Scrambled Eggs	15
Egg Salad with Capers & Basil	15
Potato Egg Bites	16
Red Pepper Broccoli Egg Bites	16
Breakfast Egg White Shrimp Muffin Cups	17
Mini Cheese and Ham Frittatas	17
Healthy Bacon Potato Egg Breakfast Casserole	18
French Toast Casserole	18
French Toast Soufflé	19
Hot Cross Buns	19
Poached Eggs with Braised Onions and Peppers	20
Banana Almond Milk Smoothie	20
Nettle Soup	21
Broccoli Casserole	21
No-Bake Brownies	22
Buttermilk Cereal	22
Butternut Cream Soup	23
Chia Almond Pudding	23
Chia-Pudding with Papaya	24

Dal soup with carrots and lentils	24
Mixed Berry Smoothie	25
Green Smoothie	25
Applesauce	26
Oat milk	26
Apple Juice	27
Black tea	27
Cranberry Juice	27

Chapter 5
Lunch Recipes — 28

Grilled BLT Pizza	29
Grilled Scallions and Tuna with Tomatoes	29
Chicken Cutlets with Sautéed Tomato	30
Lamb Tacos with Feta	30
Slow-Cooker Potato and Chicken Curry	31
Chicken Curry	31
One-Pot Chicken Thighs Curry and Cilantro Rice	32
Linguine Carbonara and Cauliflower	32
Pasta Carbonara	33
Halibut with Tomatoes and Spicy Squash	33
Spicy Shrimp and Corn with Quesadillas	34
Barbecue Beef Stir-Fry	34
Chicken Saffron Rice Pilaf	35
Stir-Fry Ground Chicken and Green Beans	35
Stewed Lamb	36
Pulled Chicken Salad	36
Lemongrass Beef	37
Beetroot Carrot Salad	37
Crunchy Maple Sweet Potatoes	38
Veggie Bowl	38

Chapter 6
Dinner Recipes — 39

Sheet Pan Vegetables and Pesto Chicken	40
Chicken in the Orange Sauce	40
Oven Roasted Potatoes and Smoked Paprika	41
Spaghetti Carbonara	41
Fried Gnocchi with Parmesan & Garlic	42
Sweet Potato Roasted Slices with Cilantro Pesto	42
Scallion Dinner Pancake Pierogies	43
Nigella Lawson's Turkey Thai Meatballs	44
Roasted Shrimps Scampi	45
Tartiflette	45
Fresh Herb, Goat Cheese, and Potato Frittata	46
Grilled Pear Cheddar Pockets	46
Chicken and Apple Kale Wraps	47
Cauliflower Rice Pilaf	47
Fresh Herb and Lemon Bulgur Pilaf	48
Corn Chowder	48
Strawberry and Rhubarb Soup	49
Chicken Sandwiches	49
Tex-Mex Bean Tostadas	50
Olive Dip	50
Omelet with Tomatoes	51
Parmesan Meatballs with Tomato Sauce	51
Quark Bowl with Psyllium	52
Cottage Cheese Breakfast with Mango	52
Rye bun	53
Beetroot Salad with Wholemeal Bread	53
Homemade Kefir	54
Smoothie with Strawberries and Barley Grass	54

Smoothie with Mango, Grapefruit and Parsley	55
Smoothie with Spinach and Strawberries	55
Asparagus salad with chicken	55

Chapter 7
Salads and Wraps — 56

Quinoa & Chickpea Grain Bowl	57
Green Salad with Hummus & Pita Bread	57
Green Salad with Beets & Edamame	58
Classic Mason jar Cobb Salad	58
Green Salad with Chickpeas	59
Stuffed Avocados Chicken Salad	59
Apple & Chicken Kale Wraps	60
Greek Edamame Salad	60
Spring Roll Salad	61
Turkey Kale Wraps	61
Shrimp & Avocado Chopped Salad	62
Green Goddess Chicken Salad	62
Chicken Club Wraps	63
Mediterranean Antipasto Tuna Salad	63
The Cobb Salad	64
Power Salad	64
Healthy Shrimp Artichoke Green Salad	65
Chicken Milanese and Arugula Salad	65
Crunchy Lettuce Chicken Wraps	66
Buttermilk Chicken with Tomato Salad	66

Chapter 8
Soups — 67

Roasted Thai Butternut Squash Soup	68
Coriander & Carrot soup	68
Clear and Healthy Soup	69
Stilton & Broccoli Soup	69
Celery soup	70
Pink Tea	70
Chicken Soup	71
Pea, Cucumber & Lettuce soup	71
Fat-Free Broth	72
Fish and Shrimp Broth	72
Chicken Bone healthy Broth	73
Beef Bone Mineral Rich Broth	73
Red Lentil Lemon Soup	74
Hazelnut, Celeriac, & Truffle Soup	74
Fennel, Leek, & Potato Soup with the Cashel Blue Cheese	75
Broccoli & Leek soup with cheesy scones	75
Roasted Sweet Potato, Red Pepper and Smoked Paprika Soup	76
Ginger Lemongrass Chicken Broth	76
Mulligatawny soup	77
Miso Soup	77
Sage & Butternut Squash Soup	78
Potato & Minty Pea Soup	78
Cauliflower & Spiced parsnip soup	79
Spiced Moroccan cauliflower and almond soup	79
Gruyere, Broccoli & chorizo soup	80
Tomato & Carrot soup	80
Spinach Soup	81
Cardamom & Lentil soup	81
Curried parsnip, lentil, & apple soup	81

Chapter 9
Snacks — 82

Sweet Potato Fries	83

Ale Pie and Steak with Mushrooms	83
Baked Sweet Potato	83
Roasted Honey Parsnips	84
Crispy Roasted Potatoes	84
Sweet Potatoes Soup with Ginger and Miso	84
Lime-Cilantro Sardine Salad into Avocado Halves	85
Ricotta & Cannellini Salad	85
3-Ingredient Sugar-Free Gelatin	85
Cranberry Kombucha Jell-O	85
Strawberry Gummies	85
Fruity Jell-O Stars	86
Plum and Nectarine Gelatin Pudding	86
Homemade Lemon Gelatin	86
Sour Blueberry Gummies	86
Sugar-Free Cinnamon Jelly	87
Bean and Tomato Salad	87
String Bean Potato Salad	87
Cucumber Peach Salad	87
Strawberry & Apple Salad	87
Bean and Couscous Salad	88
Asian Chicken Salad	88
Almond Salad	88
Vegetarian Nuttolene Salad	88
Nutty Green Salad	88

Chapter 10
Desserts 89

Papaya-Mango Smoothie	90
Cantaloupe Smoothie	90
Cantaloupe-Mix Smoothie	90
Applesauce-Avocado Smoothie	90
Pina Colada Smoothie	90
Diced Fruits	90
Avocado Dip	91
Homemade Hummus	91
Tofu	91
Whole-wheat-Chocolate Chip Cookies	91
Good-for-You Chocolate Chip Cookies	92
Oat and Wheat Cookies	92
Oatmeal Spice Cookies	92
Trail Mix Cookies	93
White Chocolate-Cranberry Cookies	93
Oatmeal Sunflower Bread	93
Maple Oatmeal Bread	93
German Dark Bread	94
Onion and Garlic Wheat Bread	94

Chapter 11
Extra Recipes Ready In 30 Mins 95

Smoothie with Mixed Berries	96
Fruit Punch	96
Chocolate Pudding	96
Soup with Mushroom	96
Soup with Broccoli	96
Wonton Broth	97
Cauliflower Broth	97
Ginger Juice	97
Lemon Tea	97
Soup with Red Lentils and Coconut	98
Soup with Asparagus	98
Mashed Sweet Potatoes	98
Zucchini Soup	98
Ginger and Mushroom Broth	98
Ginger Root Tea	99
Gummies Made with Strawberries	99
Smoothie with Creamy Cherries	99
Lemon Baked Eggs	99
Pancakes with Banana	99
Deviled Egg	100
Muesli Muffins with Pears	100
Shakshuka	100
Salmon Fritter	100
Vanilla Almond Hot Chocolate	101
Frittata with Spinach	101
Smoothie with Banana	101
Muffins with Banana	101
Omelet with Mushrooms	102

Appendix 1 Measurement Conversion Chart	**103**
Appendix 2 The Dirty Dozen and Clean Fifteen	**104**
Appendix 3 Index	**105**

Introduction

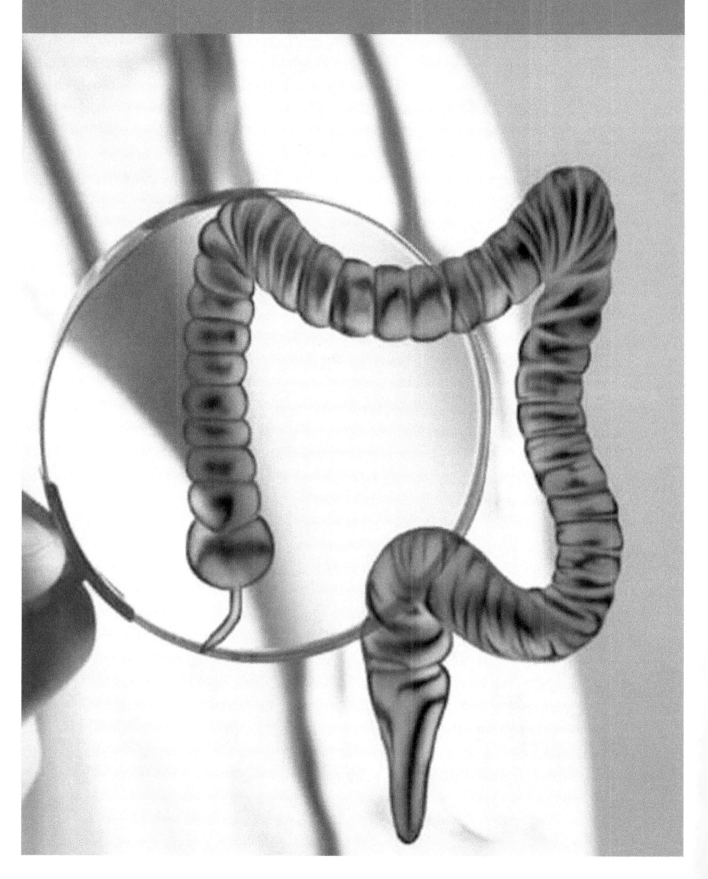

I have always considered myself an active person. In my free time, I often went jogging at the park. At some point, I even participated in the local marathon. However, that all changed in February 2015 when I experienced my first overpowering abdominal pain. I have had an upset tummy before, and this did not feel like anything I had ever felt. The pain was so strong that I found it hard to breathe or move. I was folded over and suspected there was something wrong with my body.

I visited the emergency room, and later, my doctor gave me antibiotics. However, that did not seem to alleviate the pain, and I spent several days on my back. Around April, I experienced another bout of excruciating pain, and I had to visit the hospital in an ambulance. After a CT scan and blood tests, it was concluded my pain was from diverticulitis. Having never heard of the condition before, I set to work finding out what it was.

Diverticulitis is a condition that occurs when a bulging sac forms on the colon, called a diverticulum, pushes outward, and becomes infected. In the past, Diverticulitis was common in people over 70 years of age. However, data now shows anyone of any age can get it. One of the most common habits in people with the illness is a low-fiber diet high in processed carbohydrates. In essence, the changing diets in the western world, toward more highly processed foods, are what is causing the condition to escalate.

Years of medical data now conclusively show that chronic smokers, people with obesity, and a diet high in processed food that are low in fiber are most at risk of the condition.
A diet high in fiber can help prevent the diverticula from forming in the colon. This is because fiber ensures the smoother elimination of solid waste without damage to the colon caused by constipation. When the colon walls are damaged, they thin out and are more likely to burst or bulge. Once the disease is present, diet change is the first mitigation measure. It will help to prevent flare-ups, and over time, they could become less severe.
Making huge lifestyle changes helped me deal with my condition when I left the hospital. Most of those changes involved my diet. I was given a basic set of dos and don'ts at the hospital. I knew that if I followed those basic guidelines, the chances of a relapse were low.

At first, it took a lot of work to translate the guidelines from the medical experts into real meals. It took me some time to create these recipes, but, eventually, I got them right. After consulting medical experts, they agreed that the meals introduced fiber into my diet while still being balanced.

Chapter 1: Understanding the Link Between Diverticulitis and Fiber

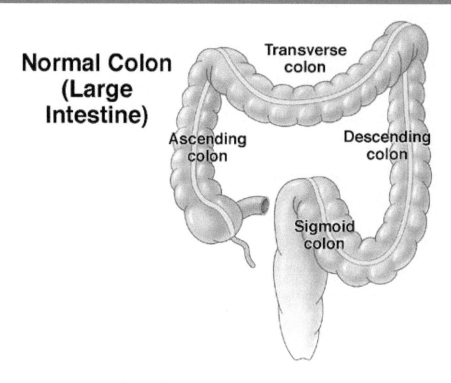

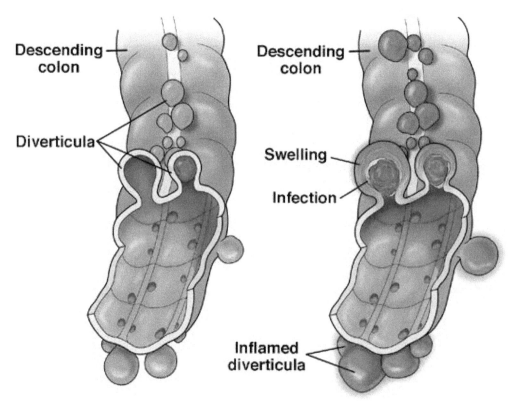

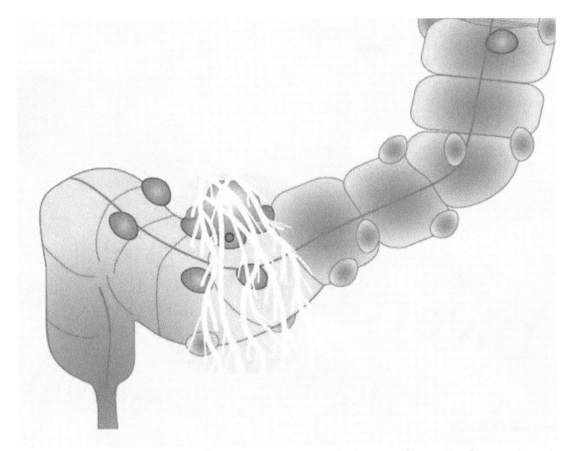

Today, all medical experts agree that fiber in the diet is an excellent means of preventing flare-ups. There is evidence to back this assertion. According to various estimates, up to ten percent of the US population will have diverticulitis by age 50. That is also the case for most other nations in the Western Hemisphere. While many risk factors are associated with the illness, one thing common in all patients is a diet low in fiber.

Numerous scientific investigations have shown that in much of Asia and Africa, where fiber-rich diets are common, diverticulitis is rare. On the other hand, in Finland, which has one of the highest percentages of an aging population, diverticulitis affects up to 50 percent of the population. Further studies show that most Finns have a low fiber intake.

Fiber, essentially plant material, is important to the digestive process. It softens the stool, which ensures it moves smoothly through the colon. Without fiber, one is most likely to be constipated, which makes the stool hard and impossible to pass. The result is additional stress on the muscles of the colon.

The diverticula sacs form in areas where the digestive muscles have been strained to their limit. When you experience constipation, it increases the chances of diverticular development. Since constipation causes pressure in the colon, it can cause an infection or inflammation of the diverticula that have already formed. The result is diverticulitis.
Luckily, the world is running with fiber-rich foods.

Risk Factors for Diverticulitis

Obesity

Obesity is having a BMI of over 30. In one study, it was found that obese people are more likely to experience flare-ups.

Red Meat Diet

A diet rich in red meat increases the risk of weight gain. When a diet is high in red meat, there is a 50 percent higher likelihood of developing diverticulitis.

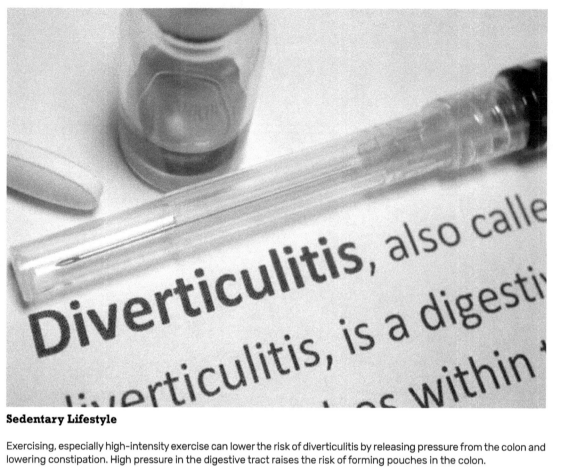

Sedentary Lifestyle

Exercising, especially high-intensity exercise can lower the risk of diverticulitis by releasing pressure from the colon and lowering constipation. High pressure in the digestive tract raises the risk of forming pouches in the colon.

Age

As we age, the connective tissues in the digestive system become weaker. Consequently, there is a higher chance of developing sacs that could burst and be inflamed.

What Foods to Avoid

Some foods are good at irritating the colon lining, leading to unimaginable pain. However, some foods will only affect certain people. Thus, listening to your body and finding out which foods trigger flare-ups is important. Generally, food that is hard to digest is likely to get stuck in the pouches of your colon. Here are the foods you should avoid to prevent flare-ups.

Seeds

All seeds, such as sesame, flax, and chia seeds, could easily be stuck in the colon sacs. Additionally, fruits with tiny seeds, like blackberries, strawberries, and raspberries, must be avoided.

Raw Veggies

Raw veggies are high in insoluble fiber, which will give the digestive system a hard time as they pass through. The result will be pain and discomfort. To ensure your body can utilize the veggies, always cook them.

Corn

Corn contains fiber and sugar content that can lead to inflammation and stomach discomfort.

Spicy Food

Spicy food should not be part of your diet. It can cause inflammation, which leads to diarrhea and vomiting. These foods can also cause a flare-up.

Cruciferous Vegetables

Veggies like cabbage, kale, and broccoli contain large amounts of fiber that your body will find difficult to digest. Eating them can lead to bloating, gas, and general discomfort.

Dairy

People with diverticulitis do not process lactose well. Even when lactose tolerant, one will experience gas, bloating, and inflammation when consuming dairy.

Greasy Fast Food

Fried, greasy food is not suitable for the digestive system in general. It causes inflammation that leads to acid reflux. In some instances, it can cause flare-ups.

Alcohol

Consuming alcohol in high doses is a risk factor for diverticulitis. It can increase the risk of getting the illness by three times. Health experts postulate that alcohol decreases intestinal motility, making it easier for food to settle in the colon sacs.

Dealing with Diverticulitis Flare-Ups with Antibiotics

A diverticulitis flare-up is a sharp pain accompanied by digestive symptoms. Sometimes, the flare-ups get so bad that one needs hospital admission. During the hospital stay, the diet is modified so that the digestive tract can heal, and inflammation will subside.

The modifications include clear liquid for several days, a short low-fiber diet, and eventually, back to normal food. In some cases, surgery and antibiotics are needed to prevent infections. However, some studies show that there is an overuse of antibiotics in some cases. It is why diet and nutrition are the most important for managing the condition, not only during a flare-up but also afterward.

Using Probiotics to Manage Diverticulitis

Probiotics are healthy gut bacteria. Some studies show that some strains can reduce the symptoms of the condition. When a high-fiber diet is combined with probiotics, it can help prevent short-term pain. The use of probiotics in combination with anti-inflammatory medication has also been shown to work. However, it is not known whether it reduces the risk of a recurrence.

Probiotics are present in fermented foods like Yakult, yogurt, kefir, sauerkraut, kimchee, miso, and tempeh. They can also be found in supplements. However, it has yet to be discovered which strains work best.

Chapter 2
Treatments and Care for Diverticulitis

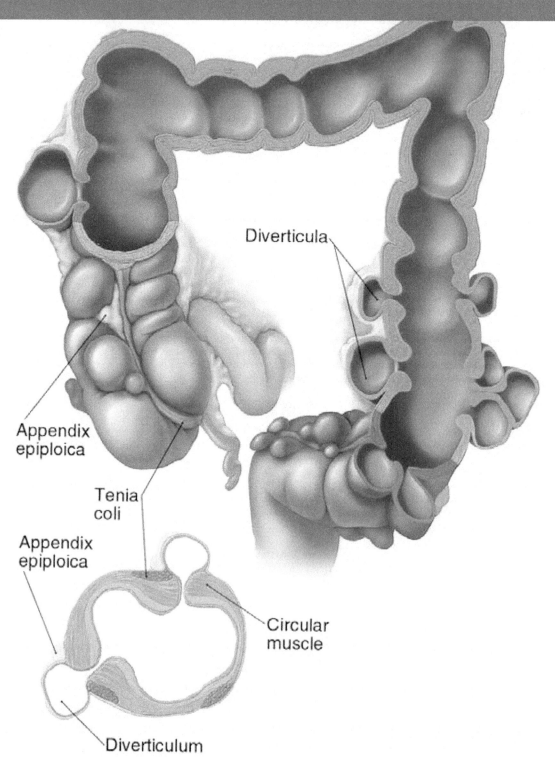

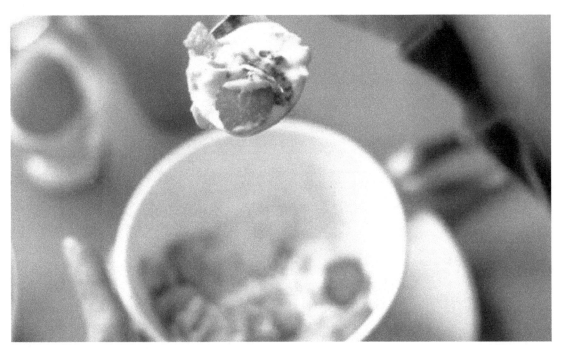

Treating Uncomplicated Diverticulitis

For most people, diverticulitis starts as a sudden wave of pain in the abdomen. In most cases, the results will show diverticulitis without any other problems. In such an instance, treatment is easy, and you will recover and go home soon. Treatment includes:

A Liquid Diet

During a flare-up, patients will be placed on bowel rest plus a diet of clear liquid. This will go on as the symptoms improve in the coming three days.

During this stage of treatment, the goal is to rest the colon and reduce irritation. A liquid diet will last for three days, giving the colon time to heal. Once it has healed, the doctor will reintroduce a low-fiber diet. This could include green beans, eggs, carrots, refined white bread, and poultry.

Pain Medication

The pain will not disappear overnight. It could last a few days because of the condition. To reduce the agony, a doctor will prescribe pain killers that will take the edge off. One of the most effective compounds for pain relief is acetaminophen. The reason for this is that aspirin and ibuprofen can cause abdominal discomfort.

Antibiotics

In the past, oral antibiotics were the first line of medication. However, new guidelines state that uncomplicated diverticulitis can be managed without them. For most people, bowel results and a liquid diet will do it. However, antibiotics are advised for those who are medically weak.

Some alternative treatments have been proposed to deal with the flare-ups. They include slippery elm, marshmallow, and licorice root. Additionally, acupuncture has been suggested to improve pain relief. However, some medical professionals note there needs to be more data to determine their efficacy.

That is different from saying one should not try these alternative methods. However, care should be taken, including advice from medical professionals.

Treating Complicated Diverticulitis

Uncomplicated diverticulitis only needs a brief visit to the hospital. However, complicated diverticulitis is different,

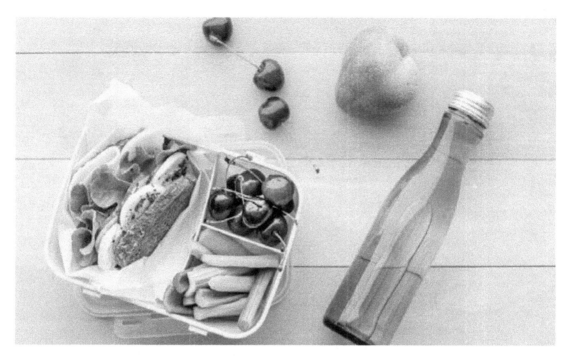

and the treatment regime may not work as well by using a few days of bowel rest and a liquid diet.

Complicated diverticulitis entails a more advanced illness. It could include perforation of the colon, fistula, bleeding, and abscesses. Such complications mean hospitalization is necessary. Additionally, there is a higher chance that the patient will need surgery.

With complex diverticulitis, the treatment could be as follows:

Intravenous Antibiotics and Pain Therapy

Complicated diverticulitis could make it hard to keep medication down. In such a case, it will be given intravenously. It ensures the medication enters your bloodstream and starts working. The process entails connecting a tube to your vein and supplying pain medication and antibiotics into the bloodstream.

Surgery

If the condition has progressed, the doctor could suggest surgery as an effective treatment. A significant reason for surgery is perforation, fistula, abscess, or internal blockage. In such an instance, the condition is so severe that there is no other solution.

Surgery eliminates any colon that is affected beyond repair. It entails cutting out the sick section of the colon and reconnecting the healthy sections. It can be an open surgery or a laparoscopic operation.

If cutting out the diseased section and reconnecting healthy portions is not possible, a bowel resection may need to be performed. It entails the creation of an opening where the large intestines can pass via the abdominal wall. The surgeon will then attach a bag to collect waste.

The procedure, called a colostomy, is not permanent for some people. If a follow-up shows that the condition improved, your colon could be reconnected.

If you have an abscess or pus pocket, it may heal with antibiotics. It could also be drained via surgery. Sometimes, a needle could be inserted via the skin to drain it.

Surgery is reserved for complex situations. However, there are many options for elective surgery for acute uncomplicated flare-ups. It is especially so when it does not always go away and keeps coming back. Surgery could provide an effective solution for the situation.

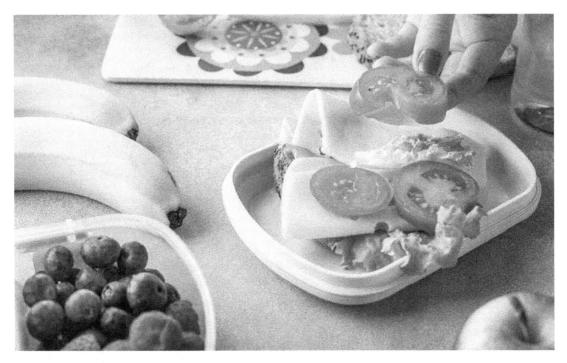

What to Expect After Surgery

One of the patients' biggest fears about surgery for their condition is that they will need to wear a bag. However, a bag is only needed in around one percent of patients that undergo surgery. Even then, the bag is temporary. Within six months, the bags will no longer be needed.

After surgery, you will remain in observations until:

- You can pass gas.
- You can urinate and defecate without assistance.
- Show no signs of infection such as warmth, discharge, and tenderness at the incisions.
- You can walk without aid or discomfort.

Once you get home, you can expect to have recurring diarrhea for about a month. It will take about three months for the bowel to attain normal status. Do not lift heavy objects during this time, as it could cause a hernia. After two weeks of leaving the hospital, you will go for a visit to discuss progress and set a timetable for your return to work and other everyday life activities. In most cases, the average is eight weeks.

How Do You Adhere to a Diet?

With the right care and habits, most people can avoid another flare-up for a decade. The right diet is essential to ensuring that you can also avoid a flare-up. Below are some useful tips on how to adhere to your diet.

Listen to the Experts

If you are trying to live healthily to manage your condition, you should always listen to what medical experts say. Following what they say can help you eliminate the condition for years to come. One expert to talk to is a registered nutritionist or dietitian. They can give you proper advice on managing the condition while getting all of your nutrients. A behavioral change expert can help to ensure smooth sailing during your change.

Learn What Works for You

No matter what the meal plans say, only choose what works for you. If a certain meal is said to be high in fiber but each time you eat it, it gives you an upset stomach, avoid it. You know your body best. What is good for another may not be good for your situation. For instance, you may have some allergy to one food, which could end up causing a flare-up.

Make Healthy Foods Part of Your Life

One of the leading causes of diverticulitis is processed foods rich in carbohydrates. The trend toward these foods is growing. To avoid the issues, surround yourself with healthy foods. Make it a point to visit the local groceries and find foods that work for you.

To avoid temptation, remove unhealthy foods from your house altogether. Even a sip of a high-fructose drink could start you on a journey that ends with you on the operating table. Keep the pantry stocked with whole foods rich in fiber and nutrients. That way, even when the cravings come, you have no option but to eat healthily.

The All-or-Nothing Approach is Harmful

All or nothing is the wrong approach to eating healthy. Try to look for foods that improve how you eat. One wrong decision should not be used as an excuse to break from your diet.

Plan Ahead when Eating Out

If you are going out, ensure that you plan. Always know what you will eat and avoid processed foods that could damage your colon. While eating in social settings, such as a wedding, have a mental plan beforehand to ensure you avoid food that could cause damage to your gut.

Get Your Family Involved

If you plan to use a diet to get your life back, always involve your family. They will provide the moral support needed to help you stick to the proper diet. Their love and support will be useful in getting you on the right track.

Get Moving

While exercise is not enough to cure diverticulitis, it helps ensure you are healthy. Get moving, and if you are already active, keep going. The pain that came with your first flare-up might discourage you from being active. However, that death spiral will make the situation worse over time. Always stay active and work out as often as possible.

Eliminate Alcohol

While medical data says you can take a bit of alcohol without flare-ups, it is not worth it. Any amount of alcohol is harmful to you at this point. Since it does not add anything to your body, you do not need it. Besides, drinking a bit of alcohol could trigger you to drink more.

Eliminate Tobacco

There is an undeniable link between tobacco use and diverticulitis. If you are trying to eat healthily, the benefits are canceled when you partake in tobacco. All tobacco products are harmful to your condition, and it is time to cut them out. The best strategy to stop smoking is to stop immediately. While you may experience night sweats and headaches, you will be on a journey to better health.

TRY THESE HEALTHY RECIPES

Data has proven that eating healthily can prevent flare-ups and manage the condition. With the right foods, you may never have to deal with an incident for the rest of your life. Eating healthily can be an enjoyable experience.

You can still get all the fiber you need while enjoying your meals. The recipes below are designed with this in mind. They are carefully crafted to give you the nutrition your body needs while helping to heal your colon.

It is not going to happen overnight. However, if you commit to eating these delicious meals, you can be sure that your condition will vastly improve. You do not need to worry about it advancing to the stages where you might need surgery. All the meals are designed to be easy to prepare while giving your body all the nutrients it needs. Besides that, they are designed for the entire family to enjoy together.

Start healing your colon today. Try one of these delicious recipes!

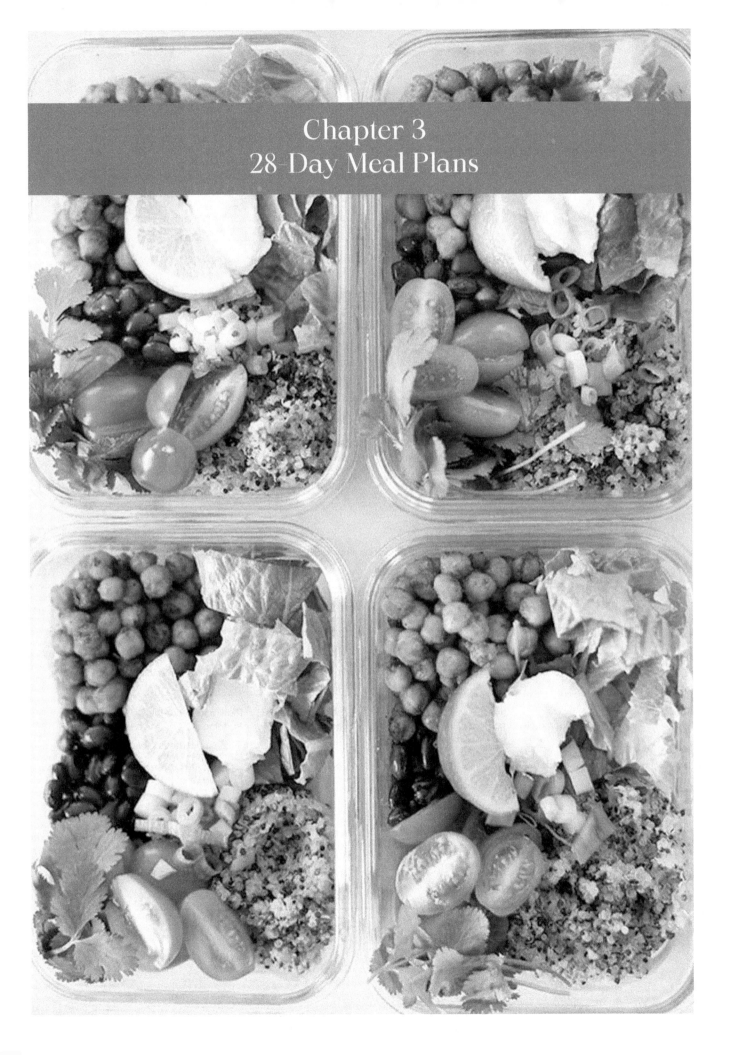

Chapter 3
28-Day Meal Plans

Week 1

Here is the following first week's meal plan for the diverticulitis diet. Try to follow the plan thoroughly to start getting the benefits of a diverticulitis diet.

Meal Plan	Breakfast	Lunch	Dinner	Snack
Day-1	Scrambled Eggs	Grilled BLT Pizza	Stilton & Broccoli soup	Smoothie with spinach and strawberries
Day-2	Egg Salad with Capers & Basil	Oven Roasted Potatoes and Smoked Paprika	Green Salad with Beets & Edamame	Baked Sweet Potato
Day-3	Black tea	Nigella Lawson's Turkey Thai Meatballs	Stuffed Avocados Chicken Salad	Roasted Honey Parsnips
Day-4	Potato Egg Bites	Tartiflette	Celery soup	String Bean Potato Salad
Day-5	Cranberry Juice	Coriander & Carrot soup	Rye bun	Bean and Tomato Salad
Day-6	Fruit Punch	Spaghetti Carbonara	Green Salad with Chickpeas	Ale Pie and Steak with Mushrooms
Day-7	Red Pepper Broccoli Egg Bites	Clear and healthy Soup	Smoothie with spinach and strawberries	Nutty Green Salad

Week 2

Here is the following second week's meal plan for a diverticulitis diet. It's the second stage of the 4 weeks meal plan that you must take into account carefully.

Meal Plan	Breakfast	Lunch	Dinner	Snack
Day-1	French Toast Soufflé	Chicken Saffron Rice Pilaf	Scallion Dinner Pancake Pierogies	Pink Tea
Day-2	Turkey Kale Wraps	Beetroot Carrot Salad	Quark Bowl with Psyllium	Strawberry Gummies
Day-3	Scrambled Eggs	Stir-Fry Ground Chicken and Green Beans	Roasted Shrimps Scampi	Plum and Nectarine Gelatin Pudding
Day-4	Buttermilk Chicken with Tomato Salad	Soup with Broccoli	Corn Chowder	Plum and Nectarine Gelatin Pudding
Day-5	Hot Cross Buns	Lemongrass Beef	Tartiflette	Homemade Lemon Gelatin
Day-6	Chicken Club Wraps	Pancakes with Banana	Olive Dip	Homemade Lemon Gelatin
Day-7	Green Salad with Chickpeas	Wonton Broth	Sheet Pan Vegetables and Pesto Chicken	Homemade Lemon Gelatin

Week 3

Here is the following third week's meal plan for a diverticulitis diet. In this stage, you already got the result of the previous two weeks' diet plan. So, follow this third stage of the meal plan completely to get a better result.

Meal Plan	Breakfast	Lunch	Dinner	Snack
Day-1	Shakshuka	Halibut with Tomatoes and Spicy Squash	Tex-Mex Bean Tostadas	Diced Fruits
Day-2	Smoothie with Banana	Fish and Shrimp Broth	Fresh Herb, Goat Cheese, and Potato Frittata	Diced Fruits
Day-3	Scrambled Eggs	Barbecue Beef Stir-Fry	Pink Tea	Applesauce
Day-4	Ginger Root Tea	Miso Soup	Chicken Milanese and Arugula Salad	Applesauce
Day-5	Omelet with Mushrooms	One-Pot Chicken Thighs Curry and Cilantro Rice	Crunchy Lettuce Chicken Wraps	Tofu
Day-6	Lemon Baked Eggs	Pasta Carbonara	Buttermilk Chicken with Tomato Salad	Tofu
Day-7	Turkey Kale Wraps	Chicken Saffron Rice Pilaf		Tofu

Week 4

This is the final stage of our 4 week's diverticulitis diet meal plan. In this stage, you already have formed a habit of maintaining a diverticulitis diet. So, follow this final stage to get best the best result in your body and mind.

Meal Plan	Breakfast	Lunch	Dinner	Snack
Day-1	Apple & Chicken Kale Wraps	Lamb Tacos with Feta	Chicken Sandwiches	Oat and Wheat Cookies
Day-2	Spring Roll Salad	Stilton & Broccoli Soup	Strawberry and Rhubarb Soup	Oat and Wheat Cookies
Day-3	Greek Edamame Salad	Stir-Fry Ground Chicken and Green Beans	Quark Bowl with Psyllium	German Dark Bread
Day-4	Scrambled Eggs	Fennel, Leek, & Potato Soup with the Cashel Blue Cheese	Homemade kefir	German Dark Bread
Day-5	Hot Cross Buns	Deviled Egg	Deviled Egg	Oatmeal Spice Cookies
Day-6	Banana Almond Milk Smoothie	Hazelnut, Celeriac, & Truffle Soup	Roasted Sweet Potato, Red Pepper and Smoked Paprika Soup	Oatmeal Spice Cookies
Day-7	Turkey Kale Wraps	Muesli Muffins with Pears	Ginger and Mushroom Broth	Oatmeal Spice Cookies

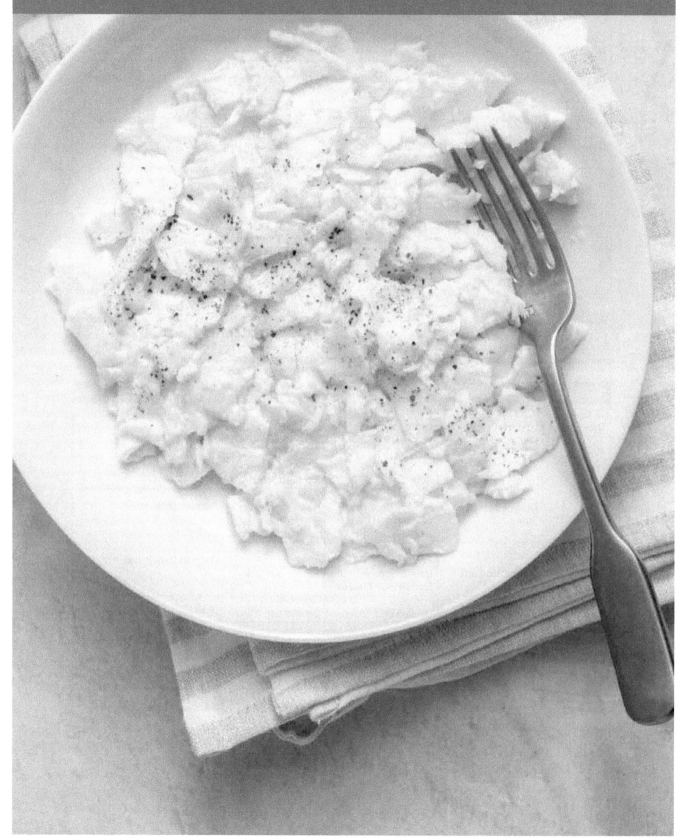

Chapter 4
Breakfast Recipes

Scrambled Eggs

Prep time: 5 minutes | Cook time: 25 minutes | Serves 2

- Some Sea salt, to taste
- 3 eggs, large
- Some nutmeg (freshly grated), to taste
- 1 tbsp. of butter
- ⅓ cup of whole milk or ¼ cup of Greek yogurt combined with 1 tbsp. of water

1. In a mixing dish, lightly beat the eggs. Season with salt and freshly grated nutmeg. Set it aside. Pour the milk or yogurt into a measuring cup. Set it aside.
2. In a cast-iron skillet (small) or other heavy pans, melt the butter over a medium-low temperature. Pour eggs into the pan after it has melted. Pour the milk into the egg bowl and stir it around to loosen any leftover eggs. Set it aside.
3. Cook, stirring constantly until the eggs begin to firm just at the bottom and edges of the pan. Stir in the milk or yogurt until fully combined with the eggs.
4. Cook, stirring regularly, for 3 minutes, or until the eggs are nearly set but still seem moist.
5. Here's a chef's trick: Turn off the heat and cover the pan using a lid. Allow the eggs to settle for about 5 minutes, just long enough to toast a couple of pieces of wholegrain bread.
6. In the steam, the eggs will continue cooking without becoming too hard or sticking to the base of the pan. Serve with wholegrain bread, compote or fresh fruit on the side, and tea or coffee as soon as possible.

PER SERVING

Calories: 199 | Fats: 16g | Carbohydrates: 2g | Proteins: 13g.

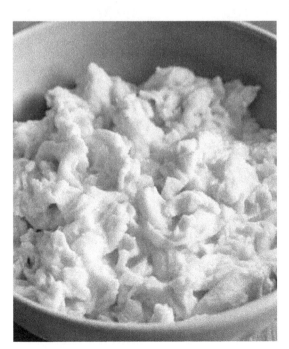

Egg Salad with Capers & Basil

Prep time: 5 minutes | Cook time: 30 minutes | Serves 2

- 1 diced celery rib
- 3 chilled Hard-Boiled Eggs
- 1 shallot (small), minced
- 2 tbsp. of Greek yogurt
- 1 tsp. of capers, rinse well
- 5-6 basil leaves (washed), shredded
- Some sea salt

1. Cut the eggs in half, then slice them up and place them in a ceramic bowl. Combine the shallots and celery in a mixing bowl.
2. Add roughly chopped capers to egg mixture together with the yogurt. Mix well and season to taste with salt. Add the shredded basil just before serving.

PER SERVING

Calories: 127kca | Fats: 1g | Carbohydrates: 3g | Proteins: 10g.

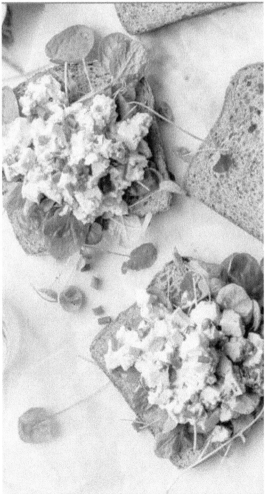

Potato Egg Bites

Prep time: 5 minutes | Cook time: 35 minutes | Serves 12

- 1 cup of cottage cheese pureed, low-fat
- 8 eggs (large)
- Some sea salt
- 2 ounces of Swiss cheese or any other cheese, shredded
- 8 ounces of peeled potato, cooked and chopped

1. Preheat the oven up to 325 degrees Fahrenheit.
2. Spray using a cooking spray 12 muffin tins well. (Silicone muffin tins are very useful.)
3. Combine eggs, cottage cheese, and a touch of salt in a mixing bowl. Toss in the potatoes. Divide the mixture among the cups. Cheese should be sprinkled on top.
4. Bake for 30 minutes or until firm.

PER SERVING

Calories: 90g | Fats: 4g | Carbohydrates: 3g | Protein: 8g..

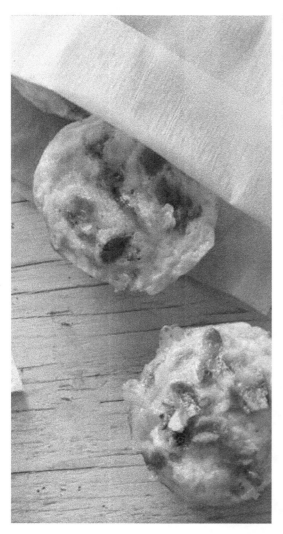

Red Pepper Broccoli Egg Bites

Prep time: 5 minutes | Cook time: 35 minutes | Serves 12

- 2 cups of chopped broccoli florets
- 1 tbsp. of olive oil
- 1 cup of chopped red bell pepper
- 6 eggs (large)
- 2 chopped scallions
- Some sea salt
- 1 tsp. of dried herb blend
- Some black pepper
- Cooking spray
- 1 cup of cheddar cheese (low-fat), shredded

1. Preheat the oven up to 350 degrees Fahrenheit.
2. In a large skillet, heat the oil. Combine the broccoli, red bell pepper, and scallions in a large mixing bowl. Season with salt and black pepper to taste. Cook for 1-2 minutes. Cover pan with 1 tbsp. Of water and heat until broccoli is barely cooked, perhaps another 1 minute or 2. Place on a platter and set aside to cool to room temperature.
3. Cooking spray non-stick small muffin pans generously. Divide the cooked veggies amongst the muffin pans.
4. Combine the eggs, salt, pepper, and dry herb mixture in a mixing bowl. Divide the egg mixture amongst the muffin pans.
5. Top each pan with a slice of cheese.
6. Bake for 15 minutes, or until well done.

PER SERVING

Calories: 72g | Fats: 4g | Carbohydrates: 2g | Protein: 6g.

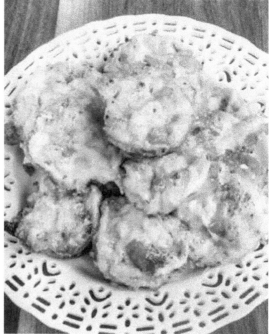

Breakfast Egg White Shrimp Muffin Cups

Prep time: 5 minutes | Cook time: 40 minutes | Serves 6

- 1 minced garlic clove
- 2 tsp. of olive oil
- 1 tbsp. of jalapeno, finely chopped
- 1/2 cup of red bell pepper chopped or sliced
- 1 finely chopped scallion
- 1/2 cup of corn
- 3 cups of spinach
- 1/4 pound of shelled shrimp, deveined and coarsely chopped (approx. 3/4 cup)
- 1 cup and 2 tbsp. of liquid egg whites
- 1/4 tsp. of sea salt
- 1/8 tsp. of turmeric
- 1/4 tsp. of black pepper

1. Preheat the oven up to 375 degrees Fahrenheit.
2. In a large pan, heat the oil and cook the garlic, jalapeño, white sections of the red bell pepper, scallion, and corn for one minute. Sauté for another minute with the shrimp, 1/8 teaspoon salt, and 1/8 teaspoon pepper. Add the spinach and cook until it is barely wilted. Remove from the heat and set aside to cool.
3. Whisk together turmeric, egg whites, 1/8 teaspoon salt, and 1/8 tsp. of pepper in a medium bowl.
4. Grease 6 non-stick muffin pans properly. Fill the pans halfway with the shrimp and veggie mixture. Pour the egg white mixture carefully over the veggies, up to the rims of the muffin pans. On top, scallion greens should be sprinkled.
5. Bake for 20 minutes or until the egg whites are completely set.

PER SERVING

Calories: 73g | Fats: 1g | Carbohydrates: 5g | Protein: 9g.

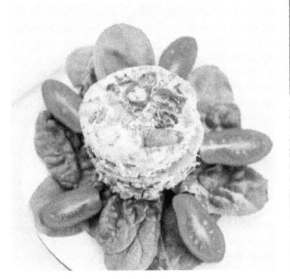

Mini Cheese and Ham Frittatas

Prep time: 5 minutes | Cook time: 1 hour | Serves 24

- 1/2 cup of finely chopped onion
- 1 tsp. of olive oil
- 2/3 cup of finely chopped ham (low-sodium)
- 4 egg whites (large)
- 1 egg (large)
- 1/3 cup of cheddar cheese (low-fat)
- 1/8 tsp. of dried thyme
- 2 tbsp. of scallions minced
- 1/8 tsp. of black pepper

1. Preheat the oven up to 350 degrees Fahrenheit.
2. In a nonstick skillet, heat the oil. Sauté the ham and onion until the onion is transparent, then take from the heat and set aside to cool.
3. Whisk together the egg, cheese, egg whites, scallions, black pepper, thyme, and the chilled ham mixture in a large mixing dish.
4. Cooking spray little muffin pans generously. Fill 24 tiny muffin pans halfway with the egg mixture.
5. Bake for 20 minutes, or until the center is firm.

PER SERVING

Calories: 21g | Fats: 1g | Carbohydrates: 4g | Protein: 2g.

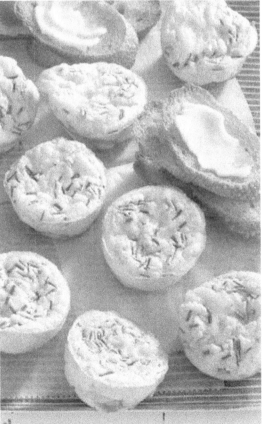

Healthy Bacon Potato Egg Breakfast Casserole

Prep time: 5 minutes | Cook time: 1 hour 5 minutes | Serves 9

- 1 chopped onion (medium)
- 2 tsp. of olive oil
- 1 chopped red bell pepper (~ 1 cup)
- 3 cloves of garlic, minced
- 1 cup of mushrooms chopped
- 4 strips of uncured chopped turkey bacon
- 6 eggs (large)
- 1 tsp. of any herb blend
- 1 cup of cottage cheese (non-fat), pureed in a food processor
- 2 cups of Yukon gold potatoes, shredded
- 1 cup of sharp cheddar cheese (reduced-fat), shredded
- 9 cups of baby kale

1. Preheat the oven up to 375 degrees Fahrenheit.
2. Sauté onion, mushrooms, bell pepper, garlic, bacon, and herb mix in a large pan until onions are transparent. Set it aside.
3. Whisk together cottage cheese, eggs, and cheddar cheese in a large mixing bowl. Add the shredded potatoes and mix well. Toss in the veggies and bacon that has been sautéed. Pour into a 9x9 square dish that has been gently oiled.
4. Bake for 45 minutes or until the casserole is set.
5. On a bed of baby kale, serve.

PER SERVING

Calories: 184g | Fats: 7g | Carbohydrates: 16g | Protein: 15g

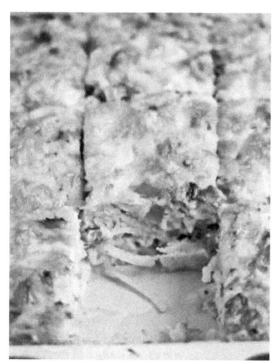

French Toast Casserole

Prep time: 5 minutes | Cook time: 1 hour 20 minutes | Serves 8

- 2 cups of half-and-half
- 8 eggs (large)
- 1 cup of whole milk
- 1 tsp. of vanilla extract
- ⅔ cup of maple syrup, plus some more for serving
- ½ tsp. of ground cinnamon
- ½ cup of pecans
- Kosher salt
- ¼ cup of raisins
- Unsalted butter for the dish
- 1 and ½ pounds of country bread or sourdough, cut in thick slices
- 2 tbsp. of turbinado or raw sugar

1. Preheat the oven to 350 degrees Fahrenheit.
2. In a large mixing bowl, whisk together half-and-half the eggs, milk, vanilla, maple syrup, cinnamon, and a sprinkle of salt. Combine the raisins and pecans in a mixing bowl. Add bread and soak for 20 to 30 minutes, rotating regularly, until it has soaked most of the custard.
3. In a greased 3-quart baking dish, place the bread in the overlapping configuration. Any residual liquid, raisins, and nuts from the bowl should be poured over. Raw sugar should be sprinkled on top.
4. Bake for 35 to 45 minutes, or until set and knife poked in the middle comes out clean. Serve warm, with more maple syrup on the side.

PER SERVING

Calories: 570g | Fats: 20g | Carbohydrates: 78g | Protein: 20g.

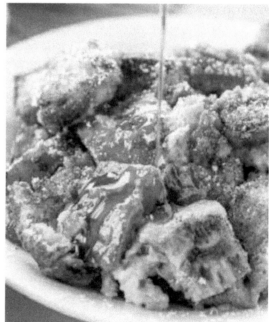

French Toast Soufflé

Prep time: 5 minutes | Cook time: 25 minutes | Serves 4

- 2 eggs (large), separated
- ⅓ cup of pure maple syrup
- ½ tsp. of vanilla extract
- ⅛ tsp. of kosher salt
- 2 tbsp. of all-purpose flour
- Some powdered sugar

1. Preheat the oven to 400°F and place the oven rack in the bottom third of the oven. Using cooking spray, gently coat 4 ramekins (5-oz.) on a baking sheet. Set it aside.
2. In a medium mixing bowl, beat egg yolks, maple syrup, and vanilla using an electric mixer onto medium to high speed for 1 minute, or until thickened. Mix in the flour until everything is well mixed.
3. Using an electric mixer onto high speed, beat egg whites & salt until firm peaks form, approximately 1 minute & 30 seconds. Gently fold 1-4th of the meringue into the syrup mixture; fold the remaining meringue into the syrup mixture. Divide among the ramekins as soon as can.
4. Reduce oven temperature to 375°F and place baking sheet containing filled ramekins onto the lowest oven rack. Bake for 12 to 13 minutes, or until puffed and brown. Serve immediately with powdered sugar on top.

PER SERVING

Calories: 177g | Fats: 2.4g | Carbohydrates: 22.8g | Protein: 3.6g.

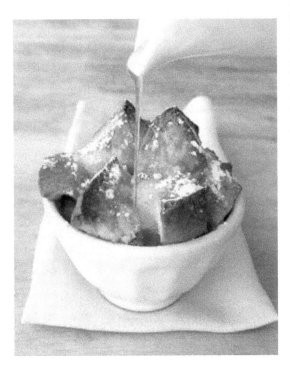

Hot Cross Buns

Prep time: 5 minutes | Cook time: 2 hour | Serves 12

- ½ cup of golden raisins
- 3 and ½ cups of Pillsbury Hot Roll Mix, yeasted (from 1 16-oz. pkg.)
- ¼ cup of granulated sugar
- ½ tsp. of ground cinnamon
- ½ tsp. of kosher salt
- ¼ tsp. of ground nutmeg
- 1 egg (large), lightly beaten
- 2 tbsp. of salted butter, softened
- 1 cup of hot water (120°F - 130°F)
- 1 egg white (large), lightly beaten
- All-purpose flour, to dust
- 1 and ½ tbsp. of whole milk
- 1 cup of powdered sugar

1. Preheat the oven to 375 degrees Fahrenheit. In a large mixing bowl, combine the roll mix, granulated sugar, raisins, salt, nutmeg, cinnamon, and yeast (given with the mix). Stir in the butter, softly beaten egg, & hot water till a soft dough comes together.
2. Turn out the dough onto a lightly floured top and knead for approximately 5 minutes, or until smooth, adding extra flour as required. Allow 5 minutes for the dough to rest after covering it with a bowl.
3. Make 12 equal amounts of dough and roll each in a 2-inch ball. In a lightly oiled 9-by-13-inch baking pan, arrange the balls in one single layer. Cover with the plastic wrap and set aside in a warm location (80°F to 85°F) for 45 minutes or until doubled in mass. Remove the lid and brush the surface with beaten egg white.
4. Bake for 16-18 minutes, or until golden brown and hollow when tapped. Allow 15 minutes to cool in a pan on the wire rack.
5. Meanwhile, combine the milk and powdered sugar in a mixing bowl and whisk until smooth. Fill a freezer bag halfway with the mixture. Snip 1 corner to create a 14-inch-diameter hole. On each bun, make an X. Warm the dish before serving.

PER SERVING

Calories: 240g | Fats: 4g | Carbohydrates: 20g | Protein: 5g

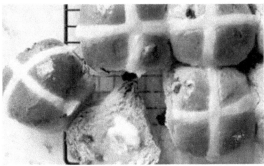

Poached Eggs with Braised Onions and Peppers
Prep time: 5 minutes | Cook time: 35 minutes | Serves 4

- 3 sliced red bell peppers
- 3 tbsp. of olive oil
- 2 onions (medium), sliced
- 1 tsp. of paprika
- 1 can of diced tomatoes (14.5-ounce)
- Some kosher salt and pepper
- 2 tbsp. of flat-leaf parsley (fresh), chopped
- 8 eggs (large)
- Country bread, to serve

1. In a large skillet, heat the oil over medium-high heat. Cook, turning often until the onions and bell peppers begin to soften, 3-5 minutes. Reduce heat to medium-low, cover, and simmer, stirring occasionally, for another 6 to 8 minutes, or until very tender.
2. Toss in the tomatoes (together with the juices), paprika, and 1/2 tsp. Salt and pepper. Cover and cook for 3 to 5 minutes, or till the liquid has thickened somewhat.
3. Make 8 small wells in the veggies with a spoon and put an egg in each. Season with 1/4 tsp. Salt and pepper, cover, and simmer over medium heat for 2 to 3 minutes, or till the egg whites are set. Serve it with the bread and parsley on the side.

PER SERVING

Calories: 302g | Fats: 20g | Carbohydrates: 15g | Protein: 15g

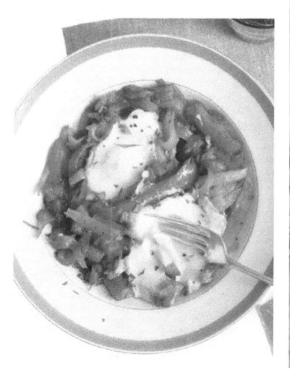

Banana Almond Milk Smoothie
Prep time: 5 minutes | Cook time: 5 minutes | Serves 2

- 2, sliced and frozen Banana
- 1 cup Almond milk
- 1 tbsp Flax seeds
- 1 tsp Vanilla extract
- 1/2 tsp Cinnamon

1. Mix all ingredients into the blender and blend until smooth.
2. Serve and enjoy!

PER SERVING

Calories: 312 | Carbohydrates: 59g | Fats: 8g | Proteins: 5g

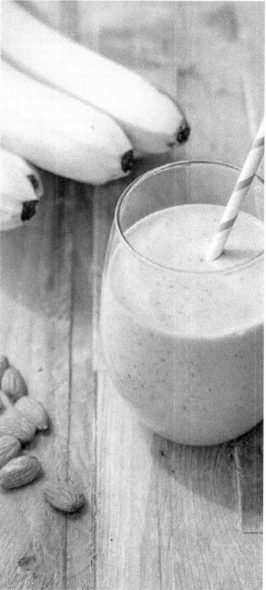

Nettle Soup

Prep time: 5 minutes | Cook time: 25 minutes | Serves 2

- 1 onion
- 2 rapeseed oil
- 3 Dinkelmehl
- 250 g fresh, tender nettle leaves
- 750 ml hot vegetable broth
- salt
- cumin
- Muskat
- coriander
- from the mill: black pepper

1. First, peel the onion, then chop into small cubes and sauté in oil until translucent. Stir in the flour to combine with the onion and oil mixture. Top up with the hot vegetable broth. Add the washed nettle
2. leaves and leave to infuse for a moment. Then puree the soup—finally, season with salt and the anti-inflammatory spices (cumin, nutmeg, coriander, pepper).

PER SERVING

Calories: 185 | Protein: 9g | Fat: 12g | Carbohydrates: 11g | Fiber: 5g

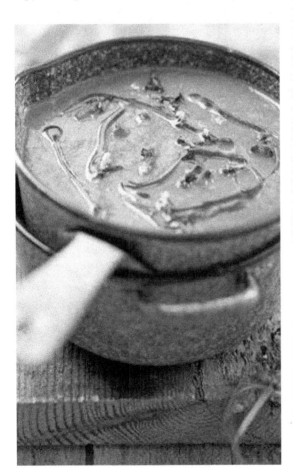

Broccoli Casserole

Prep time: 5 minutes | Cook time: 35 minutes | Serves 4

- 1kg fresh broccoli
- rapeseed oil
- 250 grams of tomatoes
- 1 onion
- 1/2 clove garlic
- 250 ml skim milk
- 3 Eggs
- 1 tbsp vegetable broth
- salt
- Pepper
- herbs
- 250 g low-fat feta cheese
- Ingredients for the tomato sauce:
- 1 can (in pieces) tomatoes
- 1/2 onion
- 1/2 clove of garlic
- pinch of sugar
- salt
- Pepper
- basil

1. Wash and chop the broccoli (alternatively: thaw frozen broccoli). Peel and chop the onion and garlic. Sauté in oil, add broccoli and 2 tablespoons of water and cook briefly.
2. Meanwhile, preheat the oven to 180 degrees (circulating air).
3. Cut the tomatoes into small pieces. Whisk together eggs, milk, and vegetable broth—season with pepper, herbs, and a little salt.
4. Place the broccoli and tomatoes in a greased casserole dish and pour the egg milk over them. Crush the sheep's cheese and sprinkle over the casserole. Cook in the preheated oven for 20 minutes. Meanwhile, prepare the tomato sauce:
5. Finely chop the garlic and onion and sauté in a saucepan with olive oil, but do not brown. Add the canned tomatoes and simmer for about 15 minutes. Season with salt, pepper, and some sugar. Season with basil if you like. Serve the sauce with the casserole.

PER SERVING

Calories: 374 | Protein: 24.2g | Fat: 25.8g | Carbohydrates: 10.6g | Fiber: 5.7g

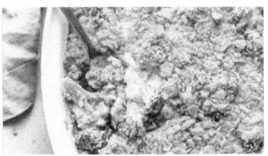

No-Bake Brownies

Prep time: 5 minutes | Cook time: 35 minutes | Serves 2

- 15 (approx. 300 g) Medjool dates
- 150 g whole, unshelled almonds
- 180 g walnuts or hazelnuts
- 100 grams of cocoa
- ½ tsp sea salt

1. A powerful blender works best for this recipe. It also works with an ordinary food processor and hand blender, but in this case, you should first chop the walnuts or hazelnuts as small as possible and then puree or grind them. If the mixer isn't powerful enough, the soaked, drained dates should be cut very small and kneaded in by hand.
2. Pit the dates, chop roughly, and soak in a bit of water for about 30 minutes. Meanwhile, roughly chop the almonds and set them aside.
3. Grind the nuts in the blender on high. They should have the consistency of flour. Add cocoa and salt and stir again.
4. Pour the dates into a colander and drain, reserving the soaking water. Add the date pieces to the nut-cocoa mixture in the mixer and process everything to form an even dough. The dough should stick together slightly. If it's too dry or not sticky enough, add a little more soaking water. Finally, knead in the roughly chopped almonds.
5. Place the dough in a shallow bowl and flatten it evenly. Cover loosely (not airtight) and refrigerate for at least 24 hours. Then cut the brownie plate into pieces.
6. The brownies will keep in the fridge for about 5 days.
7. Medjool dates are particularly juicy and aromatic. They taste slightly like caramel and are a good substitute for sugar or honey. The rich brownies taste more chocolaty than sweet with the dates filling.

PER SERVING

Calories: 439 | Protein: 11g | Fat: 29g | Carbohydrates: 29g | Fiber: 10g

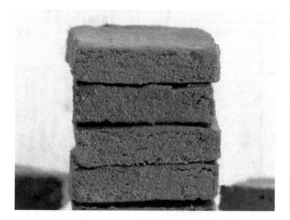

Buttermilk Cereal

Prep time: 5 minutes | Cook time: 5 minutes | Serves 4

- 150 g fresh (depending on the season) fruit
- 200ml buttermilk
- 1 tsp honey
- 60 grams of rolled oats
- 1 tbsp lemon juice

1. Wash, trim, chop the fruit and place in a bowl.
2. Mix the buttermilk with the honey and the oat flakes, season with the lemon, and pour over the fruit.
3. Mix everything loosely and let it soak for a moment.

PER SERVING

Calories: 207 | Protein: 7.8g | Fat: 2.6g | Carbohydrates: 36.7g | Fiber: 4.4g

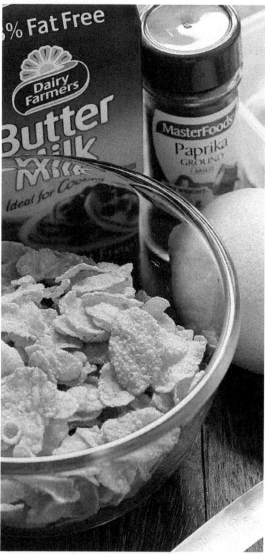

Butternut Cream Soup

Prep time: 5 minutes | **Cook time:** 15 minutes | **Serves 2**

- 1 small (about 1 kg) butternut squash
- 1 onion
- 2 tbsp canola oil
- 1 thumb-sized piece of ginger
- 1-2 cloves
- 600 ml vegetable broth
- 100 grams of sour cream
- alternatively: 100 g sour cream
- salt
- pepper
- 4 tbsp pumpkin seed oil
- turmeric powder

1. Wash and peel the pumpkin, cut into slices, scrape out the seeds with a tablespoon, and cut the flesh into pieces of about 2 cm—Peel and small dice the onion.
2. Heat the oil in a large saucepan and sauté the onion in it. Add pumpkin and sauté for about 5 minutes. Meanwhile, peel and finely grate the ginger. Add ginger and 1-2 cloves to the pumpkin vegetables, deglaze everything with broth and bring to a boil. Simmer on low heat for about thirty minutes.
3. At the end of the cooking time, remove the cloves from the saucepan. Add sour cream or sour cream to the soup and puree everything with a hand blender—season with salt and pepper. To serve, place on plates and refine each with 1 tbsp pumpkin seed oil (please never cook this fine oil) and 1 pinch of turmeric.

PER SERVING

Calories: 279 | Protein: 3g | Fat: 26g | Carbohydrates: 10g | Fiber: 7g

Chia Almond Pudding

Prep time: 5 minutes | **Cook time:** 15 minutes | **Serves 2**

- 400 ml unsweetened almond drink
- 50 g Chiasamen
- 0.5 TL ground vanilla
- 1 HE flaked almonds
- 1 HE unpeeled sesame seeds
- 2 small Kiwis
- 125 g raspberries
- 200 g (1.5%) Naturjoghurt
- 1 TL honey
- 2 TL Kakaonibs

1. The night before, mix the almond drink with chia seeds and vanilla in a bowl and let it swell for about 10 minutes. Then stir the mixture again and divide between 2 mason jars or twist-off jars, each with a capacity of around 500 ml. Cover and leave to soak in the fridge for about 8 hours, preferably overnight.
2. The following day (morning), lightly toast the flaked almonds and sesame seeds in a pan without fat over medium heat. Remove from the stove, then let cool on a plate. Peel the kiwis and cut them into wedges. Sort the raspberries, wash, and pat dry.
3. To serve, mix the yogurt with the honey until smooth. Spread two-thirds of the fruit over the chilled chia pudding and top with the yogurt and the remaining fruit. Sprinkle with the almond-sesame mix and the cocoa nibs.

PER SERVING

Calories: 364 | Protein: 17g | Fat: 24g | Carbohydrates: 19g | Fiber: 17g

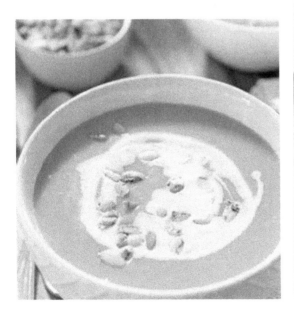

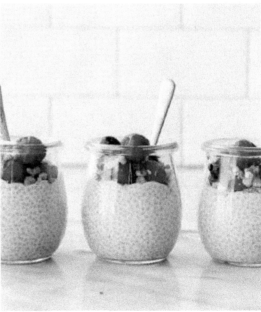

Chia Pudding with Papaya

Prep time: 5 minutes | **Cook time:** 15 minutes | **Serves** 2

- 20 g Chia-Together
- 70 ml rice milk
- alternative: oatmeal
- 1 Papaya
- 1 Spritzer
- lemon juice
- 1 linseed oil
- 1 chopped walnuts
- alternatively: almonds or cashew nuts

1. Place the chia seeds in a bowl and add the milk. They should be well covered as the seeds absorb a lot of liquid. Stir, set aside, and leave to soak for at least 1 hour, preferably overnight, in the fridge.
2. Peel the papaya and remove the seeds. Drizzle with lemon juice and cut into small cubes. Mix into the chia pudding together with the linseed oil. Sprinkle with the nuts.

PER SERVING

Calories: 460 | Protein: 11g | Fat: 34g | Carbohydrates: 29g | Fiber: 14g

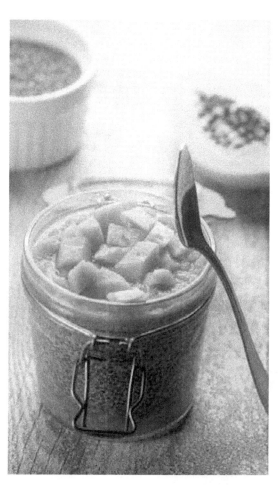

Dal soup with carrots and lentils

Prep time: 5 minutes | **Cook time:** 15 minutes | **Serves** 2

- 1 Red onion
- 200 g carrots
- 1 HE rapeseed oil
- 75 g Red lenses
- 2 THE mild curry powder
- 400 ml vegetable broth
- 400 ml Tomato juice
- Salt
- 50 g Cashew nuts
- 0.5 Bund Coriander green

1. Peel onion and chop finely. Wash, peel, and finely dice the carrots. Sauté onion in oil in a saucepan. Then, add the carrots, lentils, curry, and sauté for 2 to 3 minutes. Pour in the broth and tomato juice, bring everything to a boil and simmer with the lid on over medium heat for about 20 minutes.
2. In the meantime, roughly chop the cashew nuts and lightly roast them in a pan without fat. Take out and let cool. Wash the coriander, shake dry, pluck off the leaves and chop roughly. Mix with the cashew nuts.
3. After cooking, remove the pot from the heat, puree the soup with a hand blender, and season with salt. Arrange the dal soup in bowls and serve sprinkled with the cashew and coriander topping.

PER SERVING

Calories: 450 | Protein: 18g | Fat: 22g | Carbohydrates: 39g | Fiber: 12g | Calcium: 127 mg | purine: 35 mg

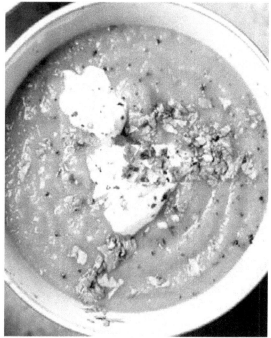

Mixed Berry Smoothie

Prep time: 5 minutes | Cook time: 5 minutes | Serves 2

- ½ cup Dairy-free Yogurt
- 12 ounces Frozen Mixed Berries
- 1 tbsp Honey

1. Add dairy-free yogurt, honey, and mixed berries into the blender and blend until smooth.
2. Pour smoothie into the glass.
3. Serve and enjoy!

PER SERVING

Calories: 171 | Carbohydrates: 38g | Fats: 2g | Proteins: 4g

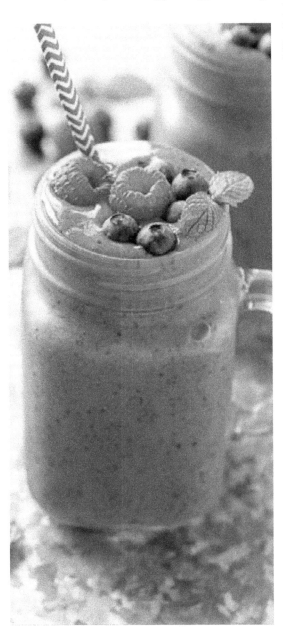

Green Smoothie

Prep time: 5 minutes | Cook time: 5 minutes | Serves 1

- 1 cup, such as almond or hemp milk Water or milk
- ½ cup Orange juice
- 1 to 2 big handfuls Fresh baby spinach
- 1 cut into coins, frozen Banana
- 1 Frozen Mango
- 1 tbsp Almond butter or peanut butter
- ¼ peeled, pit removed Avocado

1. Add water, spinach, and orange juice into the blender and blend until broken down.
2. Add peanut butter or almond butter and blend until smooth.
3. Then, add frozen mango and banana and blend until smooth.
4. Serve and enjoy!

PER SERVING

Calories: 267 | Carbohydrates: 66g | Fats: 1g | Proteins: 4g

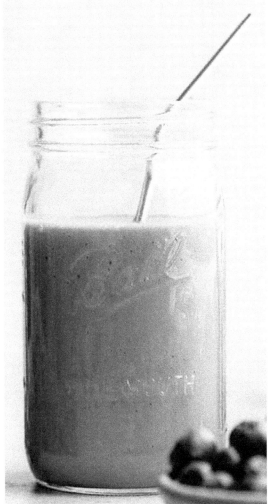

Applesauce

Prep time: 5 minutes | Cook time: 20 minutes | Serves 4

- 4, peeled and diced into small chunks Bramley Apples
- 4 tbsp Brown Sugar
- ½, juice only Lemon
- ½ tbsp Dairy-free butter
- 1 pinch Ground cinnamon

1. Add sugar, lemon juice, and apple into the pot. Place it over medium-low flame.
2. Add cinnamon, dairy-free butter, and sugar and stir well.

PER SERVING

Calories: 70 | Carbohydrates: 16.9g | Fats: 0.79g | Proteins: 0.35g

Oat milk

Prep time: 5 minutes | Cook time: 10 minutes | Serves 8

- 1 cup Rolled oats
- 4 cups Cold water
- 1 to 2 tbsp, optional Maple syrup
- 1 tsp Vanilla extract
- 1 pinch Salt

1. Firstly, add oats, water, and maple syrup into the blender. Blend for twenty to thirty seconds.
2. Strain oat milk mixture with cheesecloth or strainer over a big mixing bowl. Discard solid parts.
3. Serve and enjoy!

PER SERVING

Calories: 19 | Carbohydrates: 3g | Fats: 1g | Proteins: 1g

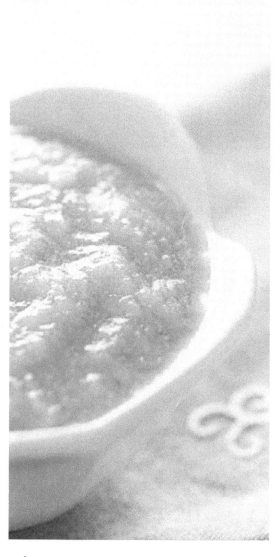
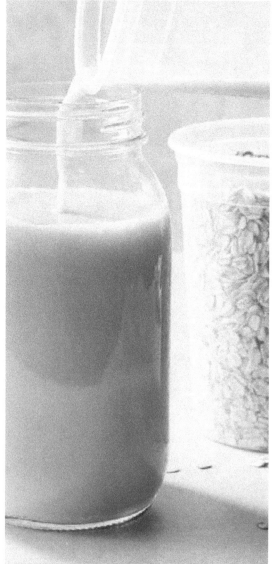

Apple Juice
Prep time: 5 minutes | Cook time: 1 minutes | Serves 4

- 8, washed and peeled Apples
- 3 tbsp Sugar

1. Rinse and peel the apples. Cut into chunks. Remove seeds.
2. Add apple chunks and sugar into the juicer and blend until smooth.
3. Serve and enjoy!

PER SERVING

Calories: 114 | Fats: 0.3g | Carbohydrates: 28g | Proteins: 0.3g

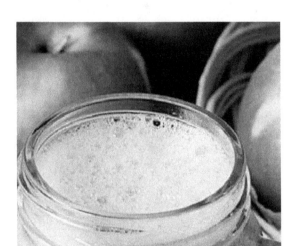

Black tea
Prep time: 5 minutes | Cook time: 5 minutes | Serves 2

- 2 cups Water
- ½ tsp Tea
- to taste Sugar -

1. Add water into the pot and boil it.
2. Then, add tea and turn off the flame.
3. Cover the pot with a lid and keep it aside for two to three minutes.
4. Add sugar into the serving cups, and then add tea.
5. Serve and enjoy!

PER SERVING

Calories: 2.4 | Carbohydrates: 0.4g | Fats: 0g | Proteins: 0.1g

Cranberry Juice
Prep time: 5 minutes | Cook time: 10 minutes | Serves 8

- 2 cups Cranberries
- 2 cups Pure water
- 1 ½ tbsp Lemon juice
- 1 tsp Honey

1. Add cranberries and water into the blender and blend at high speed for two minutes.
2. Pass the juice through a strainer or cheesecloth and remove solid pieces.
3. Add lemon juice and honey to the juice.
4. When done, serve it into the glasses.

PER SERVING

Calories: 3 | Carbohydrates: 1g | Fats: 1g | Proteins: 1g

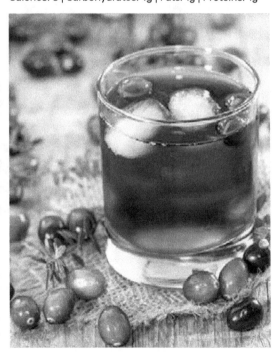

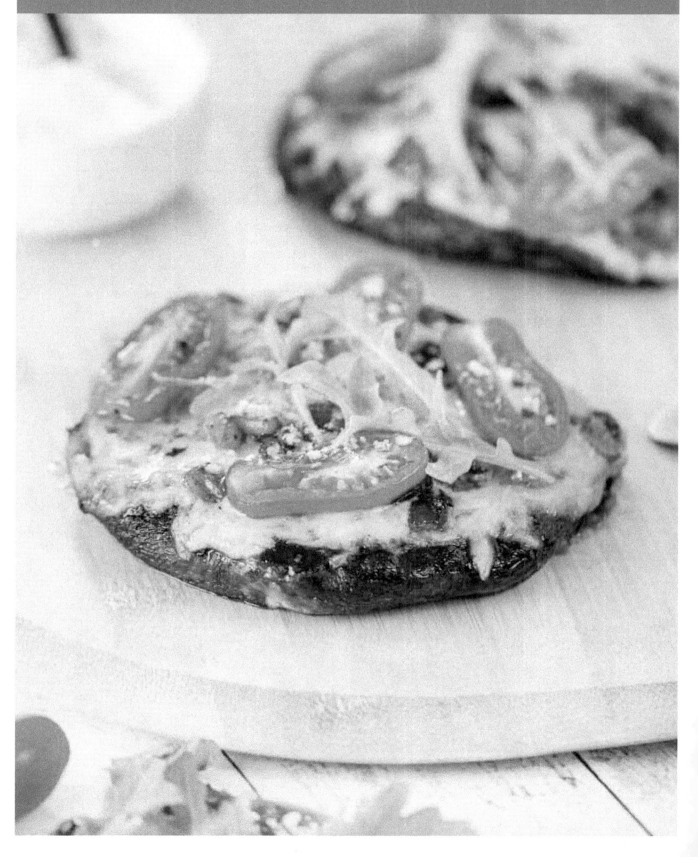

Chapter 5
Lunch Recipes

Grilled BLT Pizza

Prep time: 5 minutes | Cook time: 30 minutes | Serves 4

- Some flour for work surface
- 1 package of pizza dough, refrigerated (16-ounce)
- 3 tbsp. of olive oil
- 2 beefsteak tomatoes (large), sliced
- 4 ounces of thinly sliced prosciutto
- 4 cups of arugula or any other mixed greens

1. Preheat the grill to medium-low heat.
2. Separate the dough into two equal halves. Roll each to a 14-inch thickness on a little floured surface. Brush 1/2 tbsp. of oil over each top.
3. Place the dough, oiled-side down, on the grill. Cover the grill and cook for 3 minutes, or until the tops start to bubble as well as the bottoms become crisp.
4. Brush the tops of each slice of the dough with 1/2 tbsp. of oil and flip over immediately.
5. Continue to cook, open, until the bottoms of the pizzas are crisp and golden, 2 to 3 minutes.
6. Remove the pan from the heat and top with the tomato. Drizzle the remaining oil over the arugula and serve. Serve on separate plates after cutting into pieces.

PER SERVING

Calories: 251g | Fats: 14g | Carbohydrates: 21g | Protein: 1g

Grilled Scallions and Tuna with Tomatoes

Prep time: 5 minutes | Cook time: 30 minutes | Serves 4

- 4 tbsp. of olive oil
- A spray of cooking oil
- 1 tsp. of sesame oil, toasted (optional)
- Some kosher salt and pepper
- 4 tuna steaks (6-ounce), 1 inch thick
- 1 cup of cherry tomato halves
- 1 tbsp. of ginger (freshly grated), optional
- 2 tbsp. of fresh lime juice
- 3 bunches of scallions, trimmed

1. Using the cooking oil spray, lightly coat the clean grill. Preheat the grill to medium-high heat.
2. Add 2 tbsp. Olive oil with sesame oil (if used) into a small bowl. Brush the oil mixture over the tuna. Season with some salt and black pepper.
3. Combine the tomatoes, the remaining 2 tbsp. Olive oil, lime juice, and ginger (if used) in a mixing bowl. Season with some salt and black pepper.
4. Brush scallions with oil mixture and place in one single layer on the grill. Grill for 1 minute on each side on the grill, until cooked and slightly limp. Place on serving plates.
5. Place the tuna steaks on the grill in an equal layer. For medium-rare, cook 3 minutes on each side (4 mins. for medium and 5 for well-done).
6. Place the steaks on top of scallions on plates. Serve the tomato salad on top of the steaks right away.

PER SERVING

Calories: 340g | Fats: 15g | Carbohydrates: 9g | Protein: 42g

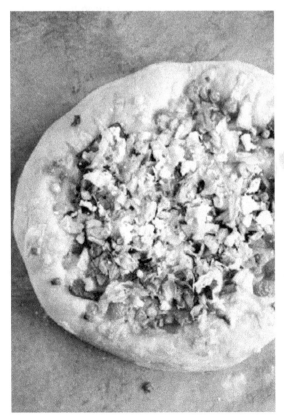

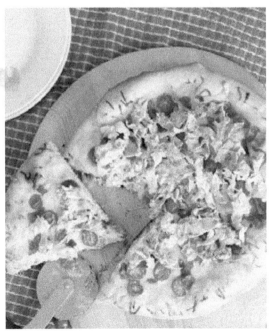

Chicken Cutlets with Sautéed Tomato

Prep time: 5 minutes | Cook time: 25 minutes | Serves 4

- Some kosher salt and black pepper
- 1 and ½ pounds of chicken cutlets, small (8-12)
- 2 tbsp. of olive oil
- ¾ cup of dry white wine (like Sauvignon Blanc)
- 1 and ½ pints of grape/cherry tomatoes
- 4 sliced scallions
- 2 tbsp. of tarragon leaves (fresh), chopped

1. Use 1/2 teaspoon salt and 1/4 teaspoon pepper to season the chicken. In a large skillet, heat the oil over medium to high heat.
2. Cook the chicken in two batches until cooked through and browned, about 2 to 3 minutes on each side. Place on serving plates.
3. Cook the tomatoes in the pan over medium to high heat, turning periodically, for 2 to 3 minutes, or until they start to burst.
4. Add the wine and cook for 2 to 3 minutes, or until the liquid has been reduced by half.
5. Serve with chicken after stirring in the tarragon and scallions.

PER SERVING

Calories: 287g | Fats: 11g | Carbohydrates: 6g | Protein: 36g.

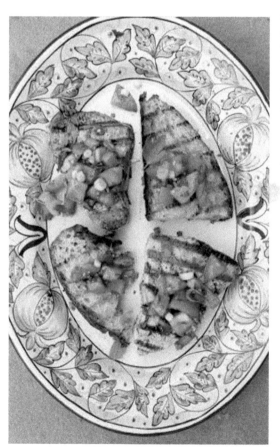

Lamb Tacos with Feta

Prep time: 5 minutes | Cook time: 1 hour 10 minutes | Serves 4

- 1 and ½ tsp. of kosher salt
- 1 and ½ pounds of lamb shoulder roast (boneless), trimmed and cut in 2-in. pieces
- ¾ tsp. of black pepper (freshly ground)
- 5 peeled cloves of garlic, smashed
- 3 tbsp. of canola oil, divided
- 1 and ½ cups of beef stock
- Pomegranate arils, Crumbled feta cheese, plain Greek yogurt (whole-milk), and fresh mint (chopped) for serving
- 8 flour tortillas (6-inch), warmed

1. Season the lamb with some salt and black pepper before serving. On a pressure multicooker, choose the sauté setting (such as Instant Pot). Preheat the oven to high, add 2 tbsp. Oil, and cook for 1-2 minutes. Cook, rotating once until the lamb begins to brown, 3-4 minutes on each side. To cancel, use the cancel button.
2. Garlic and stock should be added now. Turn the steam release handle to the sealing position and lock the lid. Cook for 45 minutes on high pressure.
3. When the cooking is done, switch the steam-release lever to the venting position and quickly release the pressure. Transfer the lamb to the rimmed baking sheet wrapped with aluminum foil with a slotted spoon, reserving 1/2 cup of the cooking liquid. Using a fork, shred the lamb into bite-size pieces.
4. Preheat the oven to broil with the oven rack 6-in. from the flame. On a baking sheet, toss the lamb with the reserved 1/4 cup cooking liquid and the remaining 1 tablespoon oil. Broil for approximately 5 minutes or until the edges begin to crisp. Remove from oven and pour the remaining 1/4 cup cooking liquid over the top. Serve the lamb with pomegranate arils, feta, yogurt, and mint in tortillas.

PER SERVING

Calories: 697g | Fats: 47g | Carbohydrates: 32g | Protein: 35g.

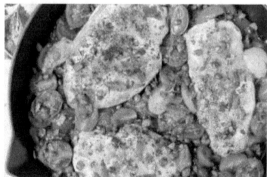

Slow-Cooker Potato and Chicken Curry

Prep time: 5 minutes | Cook time: 4 hour 20 minutes | Serves 4

- 2 red onions in wedges
- 3 peeled baking potatoes, cut in 1 and ½-inch pieces
- 3 tbsp. of chopped fresh ginger
- 2 tbsp. of curry powder
- 8 chopped garlic cloves (about 2 tbsp.)
- 1 tsp. of crushed coriander seeds
- ½ tsp. of black pepper
- 1 tsp. of kosher salt
- 6 chicken legs, skinless (3 pounds)
- Some cilantro (chopped) and basmati rice (steamed) for serving
- 1 can of unsweetened coconut milk (15-oz.)

1. In a slow cooker (6-quart), combine the onions and potatoes. In a large mixing basin, combine the ginger, curry powder, garlic, coriander, salt, and pepper. Toss in the chicken to coat it.
2. Pour the coconut milk and any loose spices over the chicken in a slow cooker. Cover and simmer on low for 6-7 hours or high for 4-5 hours, or till the chicken is cooked through and tender.
3. Serve the curry with some chopped cilantro as a garnish. Serve with basmati rice that has been cooked.

PER SERVING

Calories: 770g | Fats: 38g | Carbohydrates: 38g | Protein: 71g.

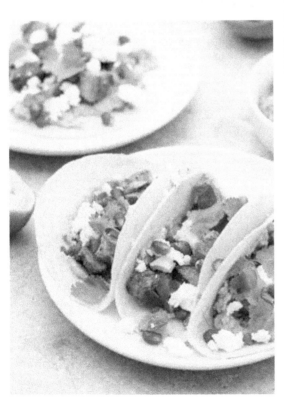

Chicken Curry

Prep time: 5 minutes | Cook time: 35 minutes | Serves 4

- 1 pound of skinless, boneless chicken breasts
- 1 cup of white rice
- 2 tbsp. of curry powder
- 2 tbsp. of olive oil
- ¼ tsp. of ground cinnamon
- 1 yellow onion (medium), thinly sliced
- 1 and ½ cups of chicken broth (low-sodium)
- 2 zucchini (medium), thinly sliced
- 1 and ½ cups of heavy cream
- ¼ tsp. of black pepper
- 1 and ½ tsp. of kosher salt
- ¼ cup of almonds (1 ounce), roughly chopped
- ½ cup of basil leaves (fresh), torn

1. Follow the package instructions for cooking the rice.
2. Clean the chicken by rinsing it and patting it dry using paper towels. Place it in a bowl and cut it in 1-inch pieces. Toss in the curry powder and cinnamon, then put aside.
3. In a large skillet, heat 1 tbsp. Oil over medium heat. Cook for 3 to 5 minutes, or until the zucchini and onion are softened. Place on a platter to cool.
4. In the same skillet, heat the remaining oil. Cook for 5 minutes, or until the chicken is browned on both sides.
5. Combine the broth, salt, cream, and pepper in a mixing bowl. Bring to a low boil, then reduce to low heat. Return the veggies to the skillet and simmer for 5 to 7 minutes, or until chicken is cooked through.
6. Distribute the rice amongst the bowls. Sprinkle the almonds and basil on top of the chicken curry.

PER SERVING

Calories: 591g | Fats: 46g | Carbohydrates: 14g | Protein: 34g.

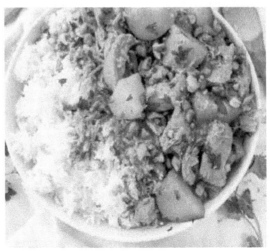

One Pot Chicken Thighs Curry and Cilantro Rice

Prep time: 5 minutes | Cook time: 35 minutes | Serves 6

- 2 pounds of skinless, boneless, trimmed chicken thighs, patted dry
- 3 tbsp. of canola oil, divided
- 2 tbsp. of curry powder
- 1 small bunch of fresh cilantro
- 2 tsp. of kosher salt, divided
- 1 shallot (large), sliced
- 1 cup of jasmine rice, rinsed
- 1 well-shaken can of coconut milk (13.66-oz.), stirred, and divided
- 3 tbsp. of creamy peanut butter
- 1 tbsp. of soy sauce or tamari
- 4 tsp. of lime juice, fresh (from 1 lime)
- Sliced cucumber to serve
- 1 tsp. of light brown sugar

1. In a big, high-sided pan with a cover, heat 1 and 1/2 tablespoons oil over medium-high heat. Curry powder & 1 and 1/2 tablespoons salt are used to season the chicken. Cook half of the chicken for 2 minutes on each side, turning once until browned. Place on a platter to cool. Using the remaining 1 and 1/2 tablespoons oil and chicken, repeat the process.
2. Set aside cilantro leaves and chop the cilantro stems to equal 1/4 cup. Raise the heat to medium-high. Cook, turning often, for 30 seconds after adding the cilantro stems and shallot. Scrape off any browned parts before adding 1 and 1/2 cup coconut milk, 1/4 cup water, and the remaining 1/2 teaspoon salt. Bring the rice and chicken to a boil. Reduce the heat to a medium-low setting. Cook, covered, for 12 minutes or until rice is soft and liquid has been absorbed. Remove from the heat and set aside to steam for 5 minutes, covered.
3. Meanwhile, in a mixing bowl, combine the lime juice, peanut butter, sugar, tamari, and the remaining 1/4 cup coconut milk. Drizzle the sauce over the rice and chicken before garnishing with cilantro leaves. Serve it with cucumber.

PER SERVING

Calories: 547g | Fats: 34g | Carbohydrates: 30g | Protein: 32g.

Linguine Carbonara and Cauliflower

Prep time: 5 minutes | Cook time: 35 minutes | Serves 4

- 4 ounces of pancetta or 5 slices of bacon, chopped
- ¾ pound of linguine or any other long pasta
- 2 tbsp. of olive oil
- Some kosher salt and pepper
- 1 small head of cauliflower (about 1 and ½ pounds), cut in small florets
- ¾ cup of Parmesan, grated (about 3 ounces)
- 1 egg (large), with extra 4 egg yolks (large), beaten

1. Drain pasta and then return it to the saucepan after boiling as per the package guidelines, saving 1/2 cup of the cooking water.
2. Meanwhile, in a big skillet over medium heat, cook the pancetta, stirring periodically, until crisp, about 8 to 10 minutes. Remove to a platter and set aside the skillet.
3. To the drippings inside the pan, add the oil, 1/2 cup water, cauliflower, 3/4 tsp. Salt, and 1/2 tsp. Pepper. Increase the heat to medium to high and cook, with a cover, for 4 to 5 minutes, or till the water has gone and cauliflower is nearly soft.
4. Uncover the cauliflower, then cook for another 4 to 6 minutes, stirring periodically, until soft and golden brown.
5. Toss the pasta with the cauliflower, egg, pancetta, Parmesan, egg yolks, and 1/4 cup of the leftover cooking water (adding more of the cooking water as required to loosen the sauce). Add black pepper to taste.

PER SERVING

Calories: 615g | Fats: 26g | Carbohydrates: 68g | Protein: 29g.

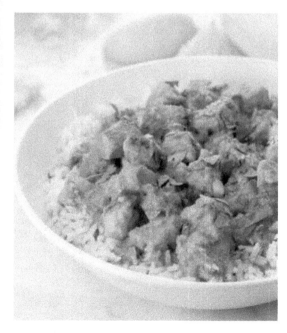

Pasta Carbonara

Prep time: 5 minutes | Cook time: 30 minutes | Serves 4

- 8 ounces of bacon, diced
- 1 pound of dry linguine
- 1 yellow onion (small), finely chopped
- 1 cup of grated Parmesan (4 ounces), plus some more for garnishing
- 3 egg yolks (large)
- ¾ tsp. of black pepper

1. Follow the package instructions for cooking the linguine. Return the pasta to the saucepan after draining, reserving 1/2 cups of the cooking water.
2. Meanwhile, cook the bacon in a pan over medium-high heat until crisp. Place on a platter lined with paper towels. All except 2 tbsp. The drippings should be spooned off and discarded.
3. Return the skillet to medium heat, add onion, and cook for 3 to 4 minutes, or until tender.
4. Add the bacon, onion, and reserved pasta water to the pasta pot as fast as possible. Cook, stirring regularly, over low heat until cooked through.
5. Remove the saucepan from the heat and add the yolks 1 at a time, stirring constantly. Stir in the Parmesan and 1/2 tsp. Pepper until the sauce slightly thickens.
6. Distribute the spaghetti across the dishes. Add more Parmesan and the leftover pepper to the top.

PER SERVING

Calories: 843g | Fats: 42g | Carbohydrates: 83g | Protein: 34g

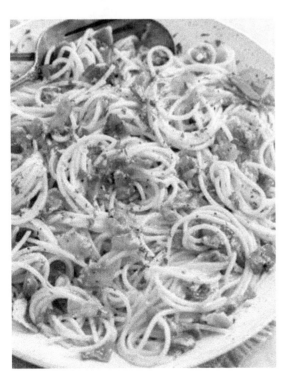

Halibut with Tomatoes and Spicy Squash

Prep time: 5 minutes | Cook time: 35 minutes | Serves 4

- 1 chopped red onion
- 1 tbsp. of olive oil
- 2 yellow squash (small), cut in 1/2-inch pieces
- 1 seeded jalapeño, thinly sliced
- 2 cloves of garlic, chopped
- Some kosher salt and pepper
- 4 pieces of skinless halibut fillet (6-ounce)
- 1 can of diced tomatoes (28-ounce)

1. In a large skillet, heat the oil over medium heat. Cook, turning occasionally, until the onion is tender, about 6 to 8 minutes.
2. Combine the squash, garlic, jalapeno, 1/2 teaspoon salt, and 1/4 teaspoon pepper in a large mixing bowl. Cook, stirring periodically, for 3 to 4 minutes, or until the squash starts to soften.
3. Combine the tomatoes & their juice in a mixing bowl. Add 1/2 teaspoon salt and 1/4 teaspoon pepper to the halibut before nestling it among the veggies.
4. Cover and cook over medium-low heat for 10 to 12 minutes, or until the halibut is flaking and opaque throughout.

PER SERVING

Calories: 297g | Fats: 8g | Carbohydrates: 13g | Protein: 41g.

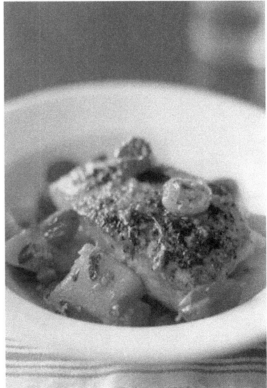

Spicy Shrimp and Corn with Quesadillas

Prep time: 5 minutes | Cook time: 30 minutes | Serves 4

- 6 scallions (light green and white parts), thinly sliced
- 5 ears of fresh corn
- 1 tsp. of fresh thyme
- 1 tbsp. of ancho or any other chili powder
- Some kosher salt and black pepper
- ¼ tsp. of cayenne pepper
- 1 pound of peeled shrimp (large), deveined
- 2 tbsp. of olive oil
- 2 flour tortillas (large)
- ½ cup of Monterey Jack, grated

1. Remove the corn kernels off the cobs using a knife. Combine the scallions, thyme, 1/4 tsp. Salt, and 1/8 tsp. Pepper in a mixing bowl. Remove from the equation.
2. Combine the chili powder, oil, cayenne, and 1/2 teaspoon salt in a medium mixing basin. Toss in the shrimp to coat them.
3. Cook the shrimp, rotating once, till cooked through, approximately 4 minutes over a medium grill or grill pan.
4. Meanwhile, spread half of each tortilla with cheese. Fold them over and cook for approximately 2 minutes, rotating once until the tortillas are crunchy and the cheese melts.
5. Cut the quesadillas into wedges after transferring them to a cutting board.
6. Serve the corn and shrimp with the quesadillas on individual plates.

PER SERVING

Calories: 310g | Fats: 17g | Carbohydrates: 36g | Protein: 30g.

Barbecue Beef Stir Fry

Prep time: 5 minutes | Cook time: 25 minutes | Serves 4

- ¼ cup Barbecue Sauce
- 3 tbsp, low-sodium Beef broth
- 1 lb, boneless, cut into strips Beef sirloin steak
- 1, sliced Onion
- 1, thinly sliced Carrot
- 1 tablespoon Oil
- 2 cups Hot cooked long-grain white rice

1. Combine the broth and BBQ sauce into the bowl.
2. Rub one tbsp of meat and let stand for five minutes.
3. Add vegetable, meat, and oil into the skillet and cook over medium-high flame for four minutes.
4. Add remaining BBQ sauce mixture and combine well. Let simmer over medium-low flame for two minutes.
5. Serve and enjoy!

PER SERVING

Calories: 310 | Carbohydrates: 34g | Protein: 23g | Fat: 9g

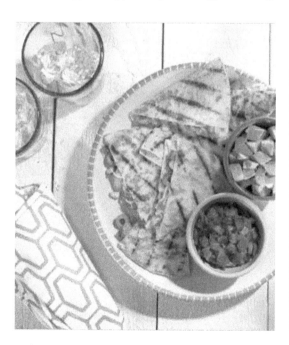

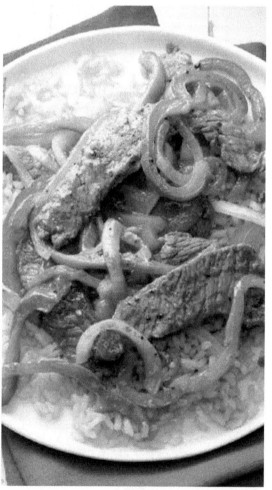

Chicken Saffron Rice Pilaf

Prep time: 15 minutes | Cook time: 30 minutes | Serves 6

- 1 pinch Saffron
- 1 tbsp Ghee or olive oil
- 1, peeled, chopped Carrot
- 1 stalk, outside parts peeled, chopped Celery
- 1½ cups Basmati rice or jasmine rice
- 3 cups, low-sodium Chicken broth
- 1¼ cups, roasted, shredded Chicken breast
- 1 Lemon
- chopped, to garnish Fresh parsley

1. Add saffron and water into the bowl and soak it.
2. Add ghee into the skillet and heat it. Then, add celery and carrots and sauté for three to four minutes until softened. Add rice and sauté until toasted.
3. Add saffron and chicken broth to the skillet, bring to a boil, lower the heat, and cook for twenty-five to thirty minutes.
4. Add shredded chicken to the rice and toss to combine.
5. Let sit for five minutes.
6. When ready to serve, add lemon juice over the rice.
7. Garnish with chopped parsley leaves.

PER SERVING

Calories: 269 | Carbohydrates: 41g | Fats: 5g | Proteins: 13g

Stir-Fry Ground Chicken and Green Beans

Prep time: 5 minutes | Cook time: 5-10 minutes | Serves 2

- 2 cups Green bean
- 1 tbsp Oil
- 1 slice Ginger
- ½ lb Ground chicken
- 1 tbsp Soy sauce
- 1 tsp Rice wine
- 1 tsp Sesame oil
- 1 tsp Sugar

1. Add green beans into the boiled water and cook until tender.
2. Drain it and put it into the bowl of ice water.
3. Add oil into the skillet and heat it. Then, add a ginger slice and fry for one to two minutes.
4. Add ground chicken and cook until no longer pink.
5. Add sugar, sesame oil, rice wine, and soy sauce and toss to combine.
6. Add drained green beans and cook them.
7. Serve and enjoy!

PER SERVING

Calories: 162 | Carbohydrates: 10g | Fats: 18g | Proteins: 22g | Fiber: 2g

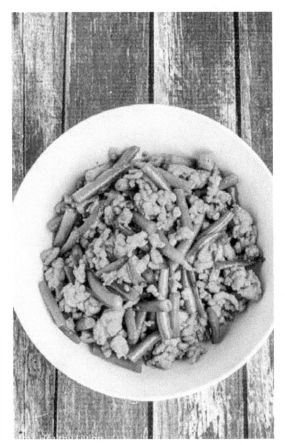

Stewed Lamb

Prep time: 5 minutes | Cook time: 8 minutes | Serves 6

- 1 1/2kg, boneless Lamb leg
- 2 tbsp Extra-virgin olive oil
- 400ml Beef or vegetable broth
- 300ml Red wine
- 80g Wholemeal flour
- 400g, sliced in half Button mushrooms
- 1 tsp Fresh rosemary leaves
- 1kg, cut into quarters, red-skinned Potatoes
- 2 chopped Celery sticks
- 2, cut into large chunks Carrots
- 1 cup, chopped Parsley

1. Add olive oil into the saucepan and place it over medium flame.
2. Cook until browned. Add stock to the slow cooker, place the lamb with all ingredients into the slow cooker, and cook on low flame for eight hours.
3. After eight hours, turn off the slow cooker and add cooled stock to the bowl to make a paste with wholemeal flour. Stir well.
4. Add flour paste and sprinkle with pepper and salt.
5. Sprinkle with fresh parsley leaves.

PER SERVING

Calories:481 | Carbohydrates: 22g | Fats: 27g | Proteins: 28g | Fiber: 4g

Pulled Chicken Salad

Prep time: 5 minutes | Cook time: 5 minutes | Serves 4

- 200g, cooked Pulled BBQ chicken
- 1/3 cup, drained, thinly sliced Apricots
- 100g Orzo pasta
- 150g, stalks removed Spinach
- 70g, cut into small cubes Cheddar cheese,
- 30g Parmesan cheese
- ¼ cup, chopped Parsley
- 1/3 cup Noodles
- 4 tbsp Olive oil
- 3 tbsp Red wine vinegar
- to taste Salt and pepper,

1. Shred cooked and cooled chicken with a fork.
2. Add cooked and cooled orzo pasta into the microwave dish. Top with parmesan cheese and microwave for one to two minutes.
3. Add apricots, chicken, parsley, and spinach into the bowl and mix it well. Then, add red wine vinegar and olive oil, sprinkle with pepper and salt, and pour over the salad. Combine it well.
4. Add crispy noodles before serving.

PER SERVING

Calories: 352 | Carbohydrates: 14g | Fats: 19g | Proteins: 29g | Fiber: 3g

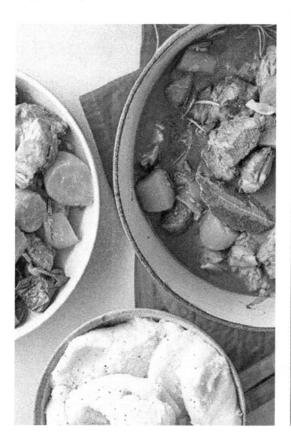
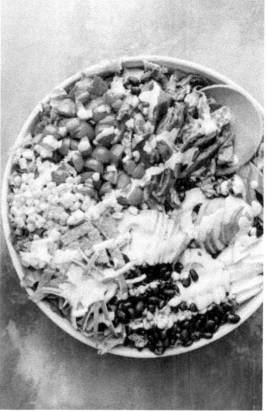

Lemongrass Beef

Prep time: 5 minutes | Cook time: 5-10 minutes | Serves 4

- 2 tbsp Sesame oil
- 1 tbsp Fish sauce
- 2 tbsp Sweet chili sauce
- 2 packets, microwave Basmati rice
- 2 tsp, shredded Coconut
- 1 tbsp Lemongrass paste
- 500g, minced, grass-fed Beef
- 1 tbsp Thai seasoning
- 100g, peeled and cut into chunks Cucumber
- 2, peeled and julienned Carrots
- ¼ cup, chopped Basil
- 1, cut into four wedges Lime

1. Add sesame oil, lemongrass paste, fish sauce, and Thai seasoning into the wok and heat it. Add the minced beef and stir well and cook for three to four minutes until browned.
2. Cook the rice according to the instructions.
3. Add one tsp shredded coconut and stir well.
4. Add carrots, cucumber, rice, and minced beef into the bowl.
5. Sprinkle with Thai basil.
6. Pour sweet chili sauce and lime wedges over it.

PER SERVING

Calories: 450 | Carbohydrates: 50g | Fats: 19g | Proteins: 21g | Fiber: 3g

Beetroot Carrot Salad

Prep time: 5 minutes | Cook time: 40 minutes | Serves 6

- 3, peeled Beetroot
- 3, peeled Carrots
- 500g, thickly sliced Halloumi,
- one tsp Fresh oregano leaves
- 100ml Maple syrup
- 50ml Fresh lemon juice
- 50g Spinach leaves
- 200g, hulled Tahini
- 100g Noodles
- 2 tbsp Extra virgin olive oil

1. Preheat the oven to 180 degrees C.
2. Wrap the beetroot and carrots into the foil and put it into the oven for forty minutes.
3. Let cool it and then cut into the wedges.
4. Add olive oil into the saucepan and place it over medium flame.
5. Turn off the flame and add oregano, lemon juice, and maple syrup and stir well.
6. Add one tbsp of hulled tahini onto the plate.
7. Top with beetroot and carrot wedges, halloumi and spinach leaves.
8. Sprinkle with crispy noodles.

PER SERVING

Calories: 206 | Carbohydrates: 34g | Fats: 6.6g | Proteins: 4.5g | Fiber: 4g

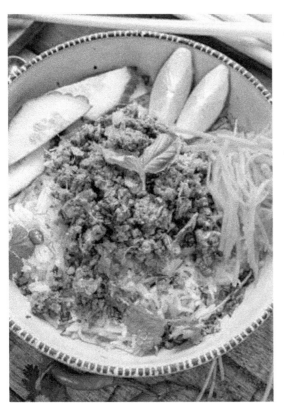
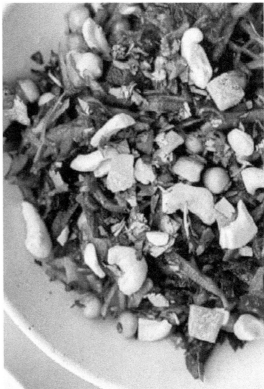

Crunchy Maple Sweet Potatoes

Prep time: 5 minutes | Cook time: 30 minutes | Serves 4

- 1 pinch Allspice
- 2 tbsp Pure maple syrup
- ¼ cup, crushed Cashew nuts
- Extra-virgin olive oil spray
- 500g, peeled White potatoes
- 1, peeled Sweet potato
- ¼ cup Plain white flour
- ½ cup Apple juice
- 1 tbsp Butter
- 1 tsp Sweet soy sauce
- 1 tbsp Maple syrup
- 1 pinch Cinnamon
- to taste Salt and pepper

1. Preheat the oven to 180 degrees C.
2. Mix all ingredients into the dish, place it into the oven, and bake for ten to fifteen minutes until golden and crunchy.
3. Keep it aside.
4. Let boil the potatoes for fifteen to twenty minutes.
5. Spray the baking dish with extra virgin olive oil.
6. Slice potatoes into chunks and place them onto the dish.
7. Add all other ingredients into the bowl and combine them well.
8. Pour mixture over the potatoes and cover with a lid and bake for ten minutes.
9. Sprinkle with nuts.

PER SERVING

Calories: 92 | Carbohydrates: 18g | Fats: 2g | Proteins: 1.2g | Fiber: 1g

Veggie Bowl

Prep time: 5 minutes | Cook time: 10 minutes | Serves 2

100g White basmati rice
6 Green beans
Red pepper, peeled, diced, and roasted
¼, sliced lengthways Ripe avocado
½ cup, sliced Cucumber
6 stems Asparagus
1 slice Tuna
½ cup, peeled and roasted Pumpkin chunks
½, cut into quarters Lemon
2 tsp, pickled Ginger
½ cup, freshly squeezed Orange juice
4 tbsp Sesame oil
1 pinch Salt and pepper

1. Cook the rice and drain it well.
2. Blanche green beans.
3. Grill red pepper and remove skin and then dice it.
4. Thinly slice the avocado lengthways.
5. Cut the cucumber thinly.
6. Drain six stems of asparagus.
7. Drain tuna slices of oil.
8. Boil the pumpkin chunks.
9. Place the red pepper in a mound in the middle of the plates.
10. Arrange all ingredients on the plates.
11. Pour sesame oil over it. Sprinkle with pepper and salt.
12. Pour dressing over the bowl.

PER SERVING

Calories: 519 | Carbohydrates: 59.2g | Fats: 28.4g | Proteins: 13.2g | Fiber: 5g

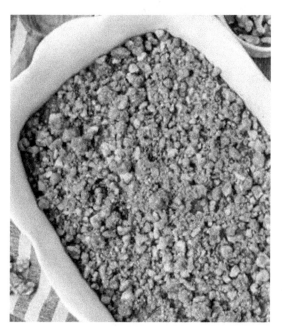
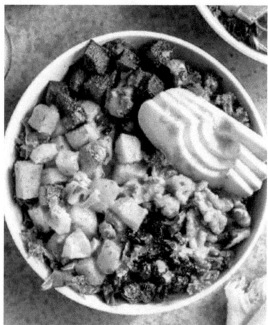

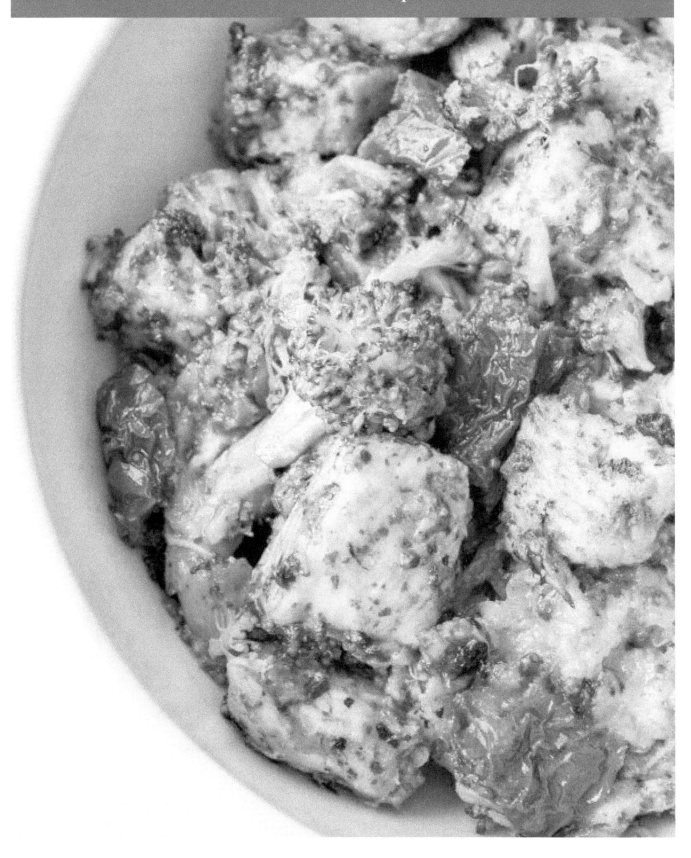

Chapter 6
Dinner Recipes

Sheet Pan Vegetables and Pesto Chicken

Prep time: 5 minutes | Cook time: 1 hour | Serves 6

- 1 lb. of skin on, bone-in chicken drumsticks or wings
- 1 lb. of skin on bone-in chicken thighs
- 1 and 1/2 lbs. of quartered baby red potatoes
- Kosher salt and black pepper, to taste
- 10 chopped carrots, in ¼-inch thick sticks
- 1 tbsp. of olive oil
- 1/2 cup of prepared basil pesto
- 2 tsp. of balsamic vinegar
- 2 cloves of garlic, minced

1. Preheat the oven up to 400 degrees Fahrenheit and prepare a wide baking sheet with foil.
2. On a baking pan, spread out the potatoes, carrots, and chicken. Season everything with salt and pepper to taste. Everything should appear like it's been dusted with light snow.
3. Combine the balsamic vinegar, olive oil, pesto, and garlic in a mixing bowl. Rub the chicken and vegetables with the mixture. Bake for 50 minutes, or till veggies are soft and the chicken reaches a temperature of at least 165 °. Place the chicken under the broiler for an extra 2-3 mins. To crisp up the skin if it isn't very golden or crispy.

PER SERVING

Calories: 640 | Fats: 38g | Carbohydrates: 31g | Proteins: 45g.

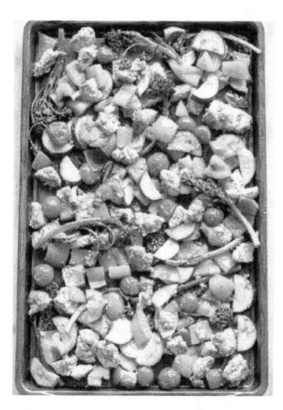

Chicken in the Orange Sauce

Prep time: 5 minutes | Cook time: 30 minutes | Serves 6

- 3 tbsp. of honey
- 3 cloves of garlic, minced
- 1 tsp. of orange zest, finely grated
- 1/3 cup of soy sauce (reduced-sodium), or 1/4 cup of regular soy sauce + 2 tbsp. of water
- 3/4 cup of orange juice, fresh
- 3 tbsp. of rice vinegar
- 1 tbsp. of peeled fresh ginger, finely minced
- 3 tbsp. of cornstarch
- black pepper (Freshly ground), to taste
- Kosher salt
- 2 pounds of boneless, skinless chicken thighs or breasts, cut in 3/4-inch pieces
- 2 tbsp. of vegetable or canola oil
- Hot cooked rice (white or brown) or quinoa, to serve
- 4 scallions, light green and white parts, sliced
- Sesame seeds (toasted), to serve (optional)

1. In a small mixing bowl, combine the garlic, orange zest honey, juice, rice vinegar, soy sauce, ginger, cornstarch, and pepper. Set aside the sauce.
2. Season the chicken with salt and black pepper to taste. In a very big skillet or wok, heat the oil over high heat. Add chicken and cook for 3 minutes, or until it begins to turn white. Add the scallions and sauce and simmer for 3-4 minutes longer, or until the sauce hardens and the chicken is nicely cooked.
3. Serve with sesame seeds sprinkled on top, if preferred, over hot rice or quinoa.

PER SERVING

Calories: 380 | Fat: 18.8g | Carbohydrates: 18.3g | Protein: 33.4g.

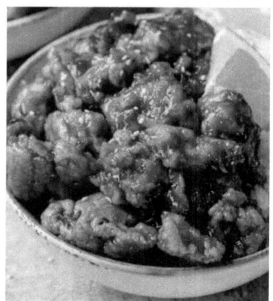

Oven Roasted Potatoes and Smoked Paprika
Prep time: 5 minutes | Cook time: 40 minutes |Serves 4-6

- 1/2 tsp. of smoked paprika
- 6-8 red potatoes (large), skin on
- 1/2 tsp. of garlic powder
- 2 tsp. of fresh chives, chopped
- 3 tbsp. of olive oil
- big dash of fresh ground pepper and kosher salt

1. Preheat the oven up to 425 degrees Fahrenheit.
2. Leave the peel on your potatoes and cut them into 1-2 pieces. Place in a mixing bowl.
3. Combine the smoked paprika, olive oil, garlic powder, and chives in a small bowl. Pour over the potatoes and toss gently until they are fully coated.
4. Place the potato cubes on a baking sheet and bake them. Roast potatoes for 30 to 35 minutes, stirring gently halfway through.
5. When finished, season liberally with coarse salt and black pepper before serving.

PER SERVING

Calories: 138 | Fat: 3g | Carbohydrates: 24g | Protein: 2g.

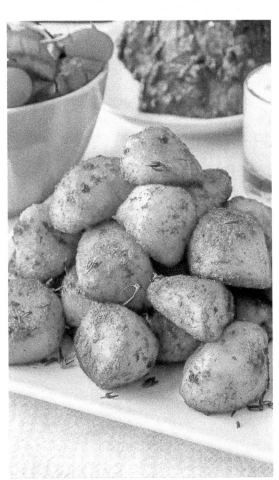

Spaghetti Carbonara
Prep time: 5 minutes | Cook time:35 minutes |Serves 4-6

- 4 eggs (large), as fresh as possible
- 1 pound of dry spaghetti
- 8 ounces of pancetta, guanciale or slab bacon, cubed
- 1/2 cup of freshly grated Pecorino
- 1/2 cup of Parmigiano-Reggiano, freshly grated
- Some Sea salt and black pepper

1. Bring 6 quarts of well-salted water to a boil (it must taste like the ocean). Cook for 8-10 minutes, or until the spaghetti is al dente. Drain the pasta and set aside 1/2 cup of the cooking water.
2. Preheat a large pan over medium heat while pasta is cooking. Add guanciale and cook for 3 minutes, or till the meat is golden brown and crispy, and the fat has rendered. Turn the heat off.
3. In a small mixing bowl, whisk together the eggs and cheeses until well blended.
4. Return guanciale pan to the medium heat and pour in half of the pasta water that was set aside. Toss the spaghetti in and stir the pan for a few seconds over high heat until the bubbling stops. A large portion of water will evaporate.
5. Remove the pan from heat and rapidly whisk in the egg mixture till the eggs thicken. The remaining heat will make the eggs, but they must be cooked fast to avoid scrambling. Thin the sauce with a little more leftover pasta water if it appears too thick.
6. Season with a generous amount of black pepper. Season to taste; based on the type of pork used, salt may not be required.
7. Immediately divide pasta into bowls and serve.

PER SERVING

Calories: 567 | Fat: 24.7g | Carbohydrates: 58.2g | Protein: 25.7g.

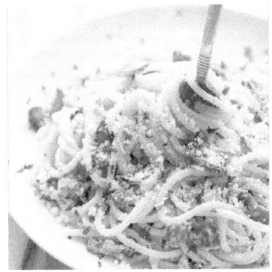

Fried Gnocchi with Parmesan & Garlic

Prep time: 5 minutes | Cook time: 35 minutes | Serves 2-3

- 2 cups of flour
- 2 and 1/2 lbs. of russet potatoes
- 1 egg
- 3 tbsp. of olive oil
- 1/2 tsp. of salt
- 4 cloves of garlic
- 1/3 cup of Parmesan, freshly grated
- 1/2 tsp. of red pepper flakes

1. A big saucepan of salted water should be brought to a boil.
2. Potatoes should be peeled and quartered before being added to the saucepan.
3. Cook for approximately 20 minutes, or until the potatoes are cooked but still firm.
4. Using a ricer, grinder, or fork, rice the potato once it has been drained and cooled.
5. Make a well in the middle of the flour or a clean, dry surface.
6. In the middle of the well, place a cooled, riced potato.
7. In the middle of the potato, make a well and add salt and egg.
8. Using a fork, combine the ingredients until they form a dough.
9. Knead your dough until it forms a ball.
10. Cut eight four-inch pieces from the rectangle formed by the ball.
11. Make a long 'snake' out of each piece.
12. Each snake should be cut into 1 and 1/2 inch sections.
13. Make an indent right in the middle of each piece with your thumb, or roll it on the tines of a fork.
14. A big pot of water should be brought to a boil.
15. Cook for 2-4 minutes, or until gnocchi floats to the top of the pot.
16. Meanwhile, heat two tablespoons of olive oil, garlic, and red pepper flakes in a pan.
17. Drain the gnocchi and place them in the skillet.
18. Cook for 2 minutes, flipping halfway through until gnocchi are crisp and browned on both sides.
19. Serve with a drizzle of grated Parmesan cheese and extra virgin olive oil.

PER SERVING

Calories: 361.7 | Fat: 10.9g | Carbohydrates: 56.8g | Protein: 9.5g

Sweet Potato Roasted Slices with Cilantro Pesto

Prep time: 5 minutes | Cook time: 40 minutes | Serves 6

- 1 tbsp. of olive oil
- 2 pounds of sweet potatoes
- black pepper and Chunky kosher salt
- 3/4 cup of shredded coconut (unsweetened)
- 2 bunches of cilantro
- 3/4 cup of shelled pistachios
- 1 hot pepper, like Thai or jalapeño (optional)
- 4 cloves of garlic
- 1 juiced lemon
- Salt to taste
- 1/4 cup of olive or vegetable oil

1. Preheat the oven up to 450 degrees Fahrenheit. Cut the sweet potatoes into 1/2-inch thick rounds. Brush with olive oil and spread in one single layer onto a baking sheet. Season with salt and black pepper to taste. Roast for 20-30 minutes, or until slightly browned and soft.
2. Make the pesto while sweet potatoes are roasting. Combine the cilantro leaves and the stems with the pistachios, coconut, hot pepper, garlic, and lemon juice in a large mixing bowl. Blend in 2 tbsp. of oil until smooth. If desired, add the other ingredients. Taste and season with salt (or garlic or acid) until you're happy. Thin pesto with water if required to make it easier to distribute.
3. When the sweet potatoes are done, put them out on a dish and sprinkle them with pesto. Serve right away.

PER SERVING

Calories: 396 | Fat: 25.3g | Carbohydrates: 39.6g | Protein: 6.8g.

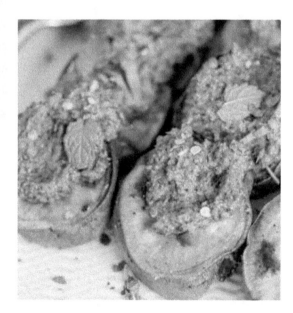

Scallion Dinner Pancake Pierogies

Prep time: 5 minutes | Cook time: 1 hour | Serves 24

- 1 pound of boneless and skinless chopped chicken thighs, in 2-inch pieces
- 2 tbsp. of vegetable oil
- 1 shallot (large), minced
- 1 piece of peeled fresh ginger (half-inch-thick), minced
- 1 garlic clove (large), minced
- 1/2 tsp. of red pepper flakes, crushed
- 1 tbsp. of soy sauce
- 1 cup of chicken broth
- 1 tbsp. of light brown sugar
- 1 tbsp. of unseasoned rice vinegar
- 1/2 cup of plain Greek yogurt or sour cream (4 ounces) (reduced-fat, full-fat, or nonfat)
- 2 eggs (large)
- 2 tbsp. of toasted sesame oil
- 1 tsp. of kosher salt
- 1 tbsp. of butter (unsalted), melted, then slightly cooled
- 1 and 1/2 cups of all-purpose flour, unbleached (6 3/8 ounces)
- 1 tbsp. of water
- 1/2 cup of scallions (minced), green parts only
- 2 tbsp. of unseasoned rice vinegar
- 2 tbsp. of soy sauce
- 2 tbsp. of honey
- 1 scallion (minced), green parts only
- 1/2 tsp. of garlic-chili paste or hot chili sesame oil

1. In a medium (3-4 quart) heavy pot or Dutch oven, heat the oil over medium-high heat. Cook for 5 minutes, or until the chicken is browned. Stir in the garlic, shallot, ginger, and pepper flakes after flipping the chicken. Cook for another 5 minutes.
2. Bring this liquid to simmer with the broth, vinegar, soy sauce, and sugar. Reduce to medium-low heat, cover, and cook for 45 minutes, or until chicken is very soft.
3. Remove the lid and check to see whether the liquid has reduced to a thick, sticky sauce. If not, continue to cook for another 5 to 10 minutes.
4. Remove the chicken from the pan and set aside to cool slightly before shredding with 2 forks or shredding with a paddle attachment on a low speed in a stand mixer bowl. (The filling may be prepared up to two days ahead of time.) Cover and store in the refrigerator until ready to use.)
5. In a mixing dish, combine 1 egg, sour cream or yogurt, butter, sesame oil, and salt. Fill a large mixing bowl halfway with flour. In a small bowl, gently combine the wet and dry ingredients. The dough may seem dry and shaggy at first, as if it would never be together, but don't worry: keep churning, and it will form itself.
6. Place the dough, along with any residual shaggy flakes, on the clean work surface. Knead for 1 minute or until smooth. Allow dough to rest for 15 minutes after covering it with the bowl.
7. In a separate bowl, whisk together the remaining water and egg to make an egg wash.
8. To make the sauce, follow these steps:
9. In a mixing bowl, whisk together the vinegar, soy sauce, honey, and sesame oil till the honey dissolves. Divide the mixture into four small basins. If desired, garnish with scallion. (The sauce may be prepared up to a week ahead of time without the scallions.) Cover and chill until ready to serve, adding the scallions immediately before serving.)
10. Parchment paper or Waxed paper should be used to line the rimmed baking pan.
11. With a knife or bench scraper, divide the resting dough into four equal pieces. Three dough pieces should be set aside and covered with a mixing bowl. Roll out the remaining dough into an 8x12-inch rectangle as thinly as possible.
12. Spoon Fill the dough rounds with 1 teaspoon filling and pickled jalapeno on top.
13. Swipe a very little bit of egg wash, just a faint touch, along the dough edge with your finger.
14. Fold the dough all over the filling onto the work surface to form a half-moon shape, or gently cup Pierogies in hand in a U shape by pinching and pressing the sides together with the thumb and pointer finger calmly but firmly close the Pierogies. Begin by pinching from the top, then moving to one of the Pierogi's "corners" and pinching around the border back to the top. To finish closing the Pierogies, repeat the process on the reverse side.
15. Repeat with the remaining dough circles and filling on the baking sheet.
16. The Pierogies may be frozen for a max of up to three months at this stage. To boil Pierogies, either fresh or frozen, bring a saucepan of water to a boil over medium to high heat (fill approx. 1 quart of water for every six Pierogies).
17. Cook until the Pierogies are floating, about 2-3 mins. For fresh and 4-5 minutes for frozen. To pan-fry boiled or fresh Pierogies, melt 1 tbsp. Unsalted butter or 1 tbsp. Neutral oil (such as canola or vegetable) in a skillet on medium heat. Fill one single layer with the Pierogies that it will fit without crowding. Cook for approximately 2 minutes on each side, or until the Pierogies are golden and crispy. Continue with more butter or oil and Pierogies.
18. You may also pan-fry Pierogies for big amounts for gatherings on a two-burner or electric stovetop griddle. Use the electric deep fryer or a big, high-sided pot loaded with 2 inches of canola or vegetable oil at least (fill the pot, not more than 1/3 full) for deep-frying frozen or fresh Pierogies.
19. Preheat the oil to 350 degrees Fahrenheit. Cook until golden brown, approximately 3 minutes for the fresh and 5 mins. For the frozen Pierogies, based on the equipment. Using paper towels, line a baking sheet. Place Pierogies on a baking pan and set them aside to cool for one minute.

PER SERVING

Calories: 266 | Fat: 18.8g | Carbohydrates: 15.7g | Protein: 8.8g.

Nigella Lawson's Turkey Thai Meatballs

Prep time: 5 minutes | Cook time: 1 hour 20 minutes | Serves 6

- 1 pound of ground turkey
- 4 zucchini (approx.1 and 1/2 pounds)
- 3 scallions
- 1-inch piece of peeled ginger (fresh), finely grated (1 and 1/2 tsp.)
- 1 clove of peeled garlic, minced or finely grated
- Small bunch of fresh cilantro, chopped
- juice and zest of 1 lime, unwaxed
- 1 tsp. of red pepper flakes, crushed
- 1 tsp. of kosher salt or sea salt flakes, plus some more to taste
- 3 tbsp. of curry paste (Thai green), or to taste
- 2 tsp. of vegetable oil
- 1 can of coconut milk (14-ounce)
- 3 tbsp. of fish sauce
- 2 cups of chicken broth
- 12 ounces of sugar snap peas
- 2-3 limes, cut in wedges
- Small handful of Thai basil leaves

1. Trim the ends off one of the zucchinis (about 6 ounces) to create the meatballs. Remove portion of the skin with a vegetable peeler in strips, then roughly grate the zucchini on a piece of paper towel: use a coarse box grater for this; if you use a fine grater, the zucchini will turn to mush. Remove as much liquid as possible from the shredded zucchini.
2. In a large mixing bowl, combine the shredded zucchini and any extra liquid, then add ground turkey, splitting it up while you pour it in.
3. Trim scallions and cut them in half lengthwise, and finely chop them, adding the white portion to the turkey and saving the green for later.
4. Add the ginger and garlic, then 2 tablespoons chopped cilantro, lime zest, crushed red pepper flakes, and salt to taste.
5. Mix meatball mixture completely but gently with a fork or hands. If you overwork it, you'll end up with thick, dense meatballs that you don't want. Shape into tiny meatballs using a heaping tablespoon as a guide after the mixture has been gently blended. If you don't start producing larger meatballs as you go, that is easy to do, and you should get approximately 30 meatballs.
6. In a big pan or Dutch oven (with a cover), heat the oil and quickly fry the chopped green portion of the onion, rotating it in hot pan. Add Thai green curry paste next, followed by the cream off the top of coconut milk, whisked into the paste over medium heat.
7. Allow the remaining coconut milk, as well as the fish sauce and chicken broth, to come to a boil.
8. Peel the remaining zucchini in the same stripes as previously, then half lengthwise, quarter lengthwise, and slice into (about) 1/2-inch pieces. Add this to the boiling pan, then carefully drop in meatballs, letting them drop in circles as you work your way around the skillet from the outside edge inward and keeping them undisturbed since they'll be extremely soft and easy to break apart.
9. Wait for pan to come back to a boil, then cover it with the lid, reduce the heat to low, and let it simmer for 15-20 minutes. Before adding the zested lime juice and sugar snap peas, make sure the zucchini is soft, and meatballs are thoroughly cooked. Check the seasoning and make any necessary adjustments.
10. Remove from the fire and top with some Thai basil or a bit extra chopped cilantro. Also, cut some limes in wedges and place them on the table for guests to spritz while they eat.

PER SERVING

Calories: 361 | Fat: 23.6g | Carbohydrates: 20.1g | Protein: 22.9g.

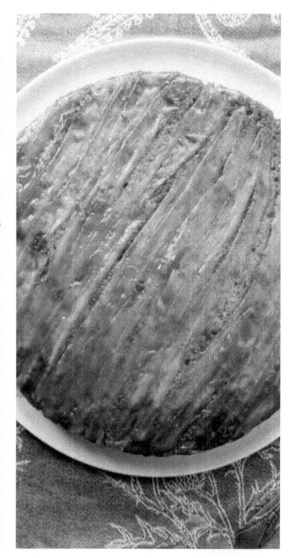

Roasted Shrimps Scampi
Prep time: 5 minutes | Cook time: 30 minutes | Serves 4-6

- 1/2 cup of unsalted butter
- 2 pounds of (26/30) peeled shrimp (medium), deveined, then tails removed
- Some kosher salt and black pepper, freshly ground
- Dash of red pepper flakes (crushed), optional
- 4 cloves of garlic, finely minced
- 1 lemon, juiced and zested, about 3 tbsp. of juice
- 3 tbsp. of Italian parsley, finely chopped
- 1/4 cup of dry white wine
- Some Lemon wedges for serving

1. Preheat oven to broil. Place a rack in the ovens top third. Thaw the shrimps under the cold running water if required. If previously thawed, rinse well and wipe dry using paper towels before transferring to a large mixing bowl.
2. In a medium saucepan, melt the butter. Toss the shrimp with approximately half of the butter and toss them to coat. Season the shrimp with salt and black pepper to taste.
3. Reduce the heat to low and add the remaining butter. Warm for approximately 1 minute, or until aromatic, after adding the garlic. Stir in red pepper flakes and lemon zest, if using, for approximately 1 minute over low heat. In a separate bowl, whisk together the lemon juice and wine. Keep warm on a low heat setting.
4. On a baking sheet, spread shrimp in one single layer and roast for 3-4 minutes, or until pink, turning halfway through.
5. Combine the shrimp, butter sauce, and parsley in a mixing bowl. Serve immediately with lemon wedges on side over pasta or veggies.

PER SERVING
Calories: 259 | Fat: 16.9g | Carbohydrates: 3.7g | Protein: 21.1g.

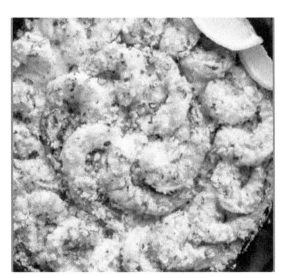

Tartiflette
Prep time: 5 minutes | Cook time: 45 minutes | Serves 4

- 250g or 8oz. of bacon lardons
- 1kg or 2lb. 4oz. of Charlotte potatoes, peeled
- 2 shallots
- 100ml or 3 and ½ fly oz. of white wine
- 1 garlic clove
- 200ml or 7fl oz. of double cream
- 1 Reblochon cheese, whole (about 450g or 1lb.), sliced
- sea salt and black pepper

1. Preheat the oven to 200°C/400°F/Gas 7 for the Tartiflette.
2. In a pan of boiling salted water, cook the potatoes for 10 mins, or until soft.
3. Drain and leave aside to cool for a few minutes.
4. Meanwhile, heat the frying pan over high heat and cook the bacon, shallots, and garlic until golden brown, about 4-5 minutes. Cook until all the liquid has evaporated, then deglaze the pan with white wine.
5. Thinly slice the potatoes and top them with the bacon mixture in an ovenproof gratin dish. Pour the double cream over the top. Season generously with salt and black pepper. On top, layer the Reblochon slices.
6. Bake for 10-15 minutes, or till the cheese has become golden brown and is bubbling.

PER SERVING
Calories: 446 | Fat: 29g | Carbohydrates: 23g | Protein: 20g.

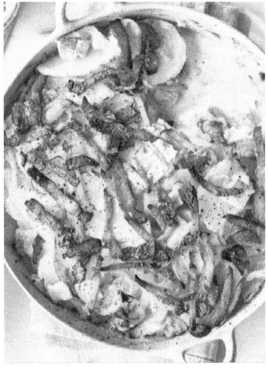

Fresh Herb, Goat Cheese, and Potato Frittata

Prep time: 5 minutes | Cook time: 35 minutes | Serves 6

- 2 peeled baby Yukon Gold potatoes, sliced in 1/4-inch thick slices (1 and 1/2 cups or 215g)
- 2 tbsp. of olive oil
- 1 shallot (medium), minced
- 2 cloves of garlic, minced
- Kosher salt and pepper
- 9 eggs (large)
- 1/3 cup of fresh herbs (chopped), like basil, dill, and chives, plus some more to garnish
- 3 tbsp. of whole milk
- 4 ounces of goat cheese (1/2 cup), crumbled
- 1/4 tsp. of kosher salt

1. Preheat the oven up to 400 degrees Fahrenheit.
2. In a 10 to12 inch oven-proof skillet, heat the oil over medium heat. Cook, stirring occasionally, until the shallot and potatoes are golden browns, about 6-7 minutes. Cook for a further minute after adding the garlic. Arrange cooked potatoes in a thin layer, equally spread.
3. Whisk together the milk, chopped herbs, eggs, and salt in a large mixing basin. Pour the mixture of egg over the potatoes in the pan, then sprinkle with goat cheese over the top. Place in oven and bake for 12 to 14 minutes, or until firm and brown on top.
4. Straight from the pan, slice and then serve the frittata, or transfer onto a serving platter, decorate, and slice in wedges.

PER SERVING

Calories: 239 | Fat: 15.9g | Carbohydrates: 9.5g | Protein: 14.2g.

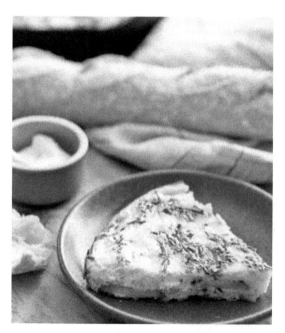

Grilled Pear Cheddar Pockets

Prep time: 5 minutes | Cook time: 15 minutes | Serves 1

- 2 tsp Dijon mustard
- ½ Whole grain flatbread
- 2 slices Cheddar cheese
- ¼ cup Arugula
- 1/3, cored and cut into thick slices Red pear

1. Spread mustard over the inner side of the flatbread pocket.
2. Place cheese slices and fold them. Then, add pear slices and arugula.
3. Place it into the skillet and cook for 3 to 4 minutes.

PER SERVING

Calories: 223 | Fat: 8.6g | Carbohydrate: 28.6g | Protein: 11.3g | Fiber: 6.8g

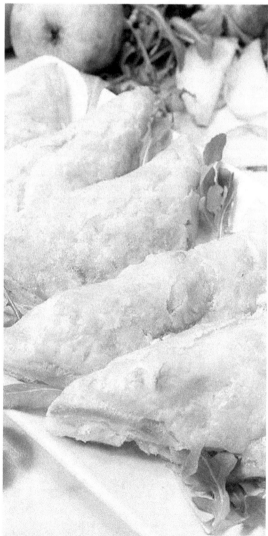

Chicken and Apple Kale Wraps

Prep time: 5 minutes | Cook time: 10 minutes |Serves 1

- 1 tbsp Mayonnaise
- 1 tsp Dijon mustard
- 3 Kale leaves
- 3 ounces, thinly sliced, cooked Chicken breast
- 6 slices, thin Red onion
- 1, cut into nine slices Apple

1. Combine the mustard and mayonnaise into the bowl.
2. Spread onto the kale leaves—top with one-ounce chicken, three slices of apples, and two slices of onion.
3. Then, roll each kale leaf.
4. Cut in half.

PER SERVING

Calories: 370 | Fat: 13.7g | Carbohydrate: 34.1g | Protein: 29.3g | Fiber: 6g

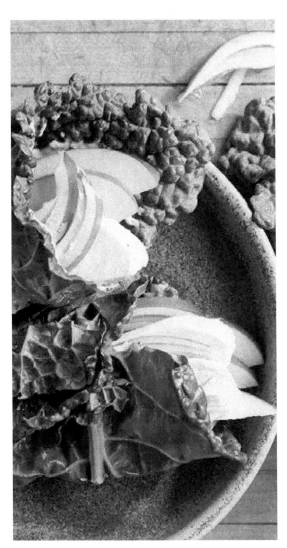

Cauliflower Rice Pilaf

Prep time: 10 minutes | Cook time: 10 minutes |Serves 1

- 6 cups Cauliflower florets
- 3 tbsp Extra-virgin olive oil
- 2 cloves, minced Garlic
- ½ tsp Salt
- ¼ cup, toasted, sliced Almonds
- ¼ cup, chopped Herbs
- 2 tsp Lemon zest

1. Add cauliflower florets into the food processor and blend until chopped.
2. Add oil into the skillet and place it over medium-high flame.
3. Then, add garlic and cook for a half-minute.
4. Add cauliflower rice and season with salt. Let cook for three to five minutes.
5. Remove from the flame.
6. Add lemon zest, herbs, and almonds and stir well.

PER SERVING

Calories: 114 | Fat: 9.2g | Carbohydrate: 6.7g | Protein: 3g | Fiber: 2.8g

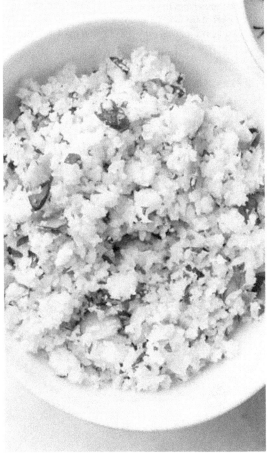

Fresh Herb and Lemon Bulgur Pilaf

Prep time: 10 minutes | Cook time: 40 minutes | Serves 6

- 2 tbsp Extra-virgin olive oil
- 2 cups, chopped Onion
- 1 clove, chopped Garlic
- 1 ½ cups Bulgur
- ½ tsp Ground turmeric
- ½ tsp Ground cumin
- 2 cups, low-sodium Vegetable or chicken broth
- 1 ½ cups, chopped Carrot
- 2 tsp, grated or chopped Fresh ginger
- 1 tsp Salt
- ¼ cup, chopped Fresh dill
- ¼ cup, chopped Fresh mint
- ¼ cup, chopped Parsley
- 3 tbsp Lemon juice
- ½ cup, chopped, toasted Walnuts

1. Add oil into the skillet and place it over medium flame.
2. Add onion and cook for 12 to 18 minutes.
3. Add garlic and cook for one minute.
4. Then, add cumin, turmeric, and bulgur and cook for one minute.
5. Add salt, ginger, carrot, and broth and bring to a boil over medium0high flame, about 15 minutes.
6. Remove from the flame.
7. Let rest for five minutes.
8. Add lemon juice, parsley, dill, and mint into the pilaf and stir well.
9. Garnish with walnuts.

PER SERVING

Calories: 273 | Fat: 11.7g | Carbohydrate: 38.8g | Protein: 7.3g | Fiber: 7.7g

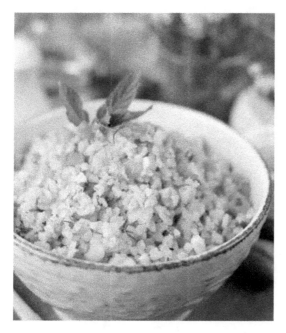

Corn Chowder

Prep time: 10 minutes | Cook time: 5 minutes | Serves 6

- ¾ cup, split Yellow split peas
- 28 ounces, low-sodium Chicken broth
- 1 cup Water
- 12 ounces, frozen Corn kernels
- ½ cup, chopped and roasted Red sweet peppers
- 4 ounces, diced Green chilies
- 1 tsp Ground cumin
- ½ tsp, crushed Dried oregano
- ½ tsp, crushed Dried thyme
- ½ cup Cream cheese

1. Rinse split peas underwater.
2. Mix the thyme, oregano, cumin, chilies, red peppers, corn, water, split peas, and chicken broth and cook on high heat for five to six hours.
3. Let cool it for ten minutes.
4. Transfer two cups of soup into the food processor and blend until smooth.
5. Add pureed soup into the slow cooker. Then, add cream cheese and whisk to combine—Cook for five minutes.
6. Serve!

PER SERVING

Calories: 222 | Fat: 7.5g | Carbohydrate: 29.8g | Protein: 10.5g | Fiber: 7.7g

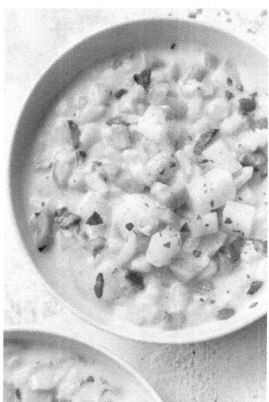

Strawberry and Rhubarb Soup

Prep time: 5 minutes | Cook time: 30 minutes | Serves 4

- 4 cups Rhubarb
- 3 cups Water
- 1 ½ cups, sliced Strawberries
- ¼ cup Sugar
- 1/8 tsp Salt
- 1/3 cup, chopped Mint or basil
- to taste Ground pepper

1. Add three cups of water and rhubarb into the saucepan.
2. Cook for five minutes until softened.
3. Transfer it to the bowl.
4. Add 2-inch ice water into the bowl and keep it aside with rhubarb.
5. Place it into the fridge for twenty minutes.
6. Transfer the rhubarb to the blender. Then, add salt, sugar, and strawberries and blend until smooth.
7. Place it back in the bowl. Add basil or mint.
8. Serve!

PER SERVING

Calories: 95 | Fat: 0.5g | Carbohydrate: 23.1g | Protein: 1.6g | Fiber: 3.5g

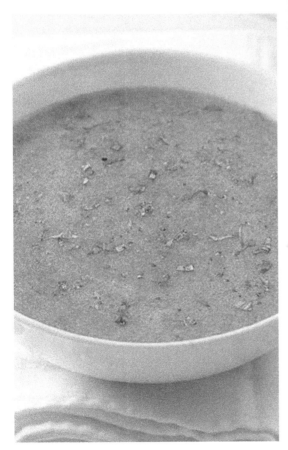

Chicken Sandwiches

Prep time: 5 minutes | Cook time: 30 minutes | Serves 4

- 4 slices Red onion
- 1, seeded and quartered Red sweet pepper
- 6 ounces, boneless, cut in half, horizontally Chicken breast
- 4, split Multi-grain sandwich round
- 2 tbsp Basil pesto
- 2 tbsp, pitted and chopped Kalamata olives
- 1/3 cup, shredded Mozzarella cheese
- ¼ cup, low-fat, crumbled Feta cheese

1. Heat the skillet over medium flame.
2. Let coat with pepper and red onion with non-stick cooking spray.
3. Add it to the pan and cook for six to eight minutes.
4. Remove from the skillet. Let coat the chicken with non-stick cooking spray.
5. Add chicken to the grill pan and cook for three to five minutes.
6. Remove from the skillet.
7. Pull chicken into shreds. Cut pepper into strips.
8. To assemble the sandwiches: Spread the pesto onto the sandwich and sprinkle with olives. Place grilled onion slices. Top with pepper strips.
9. Place chicken over it. Sprinkle with feta cheese and mozzarella cheese.
10. Then, place skillet over medium-low flame.
11. Place the sandwich into the skillet and cook for three to four minutes.
12. Flip and cook for three to four minutes. Serve!

PER SERVING

Calories: 296 | Fat: 10g | Carbohydrate: 27.7g | Protein: 25.8g | Fiber: 6.2g

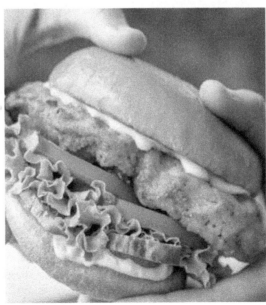

Tex Mex Bean Tostadas
Prep time: 10 minutes | Cook time: 15 minutes | Serves 4

- 4 Tostada shells
- 16 ounces, rinsed and drained Pinto beans
- ½ cup, prepared Salsa
- ½ tsp Chipotle seasoning
- ½ cup, shredded Cheddar cheese
- 1 ½ cups Iceberg lettuce
- 1 cup, chopped Tomato
- 1 Lime wedges

1. Preheat the oven to 350 degrees Fahrenheit.
2. Place tostada shells onto the baking sheet and bake for three to five minutes.
3. Meanwhile, mix the seasoning, salsa, and bean into the bowl.
4. Mash the mixture with a potato masher.
5. Then, divide the bean mixture between tostada shells.
6. Top with half of the cheese. Bake for five minutes.
7. Top with chopped tomato and shredded lettuce.
8. Then, place the remaining cheese and lime wedges.

PER SERVING

Calories: 230 | Fat: 6g | Carbohydrate: 33g | Protein: 12g | Fiber: 6g

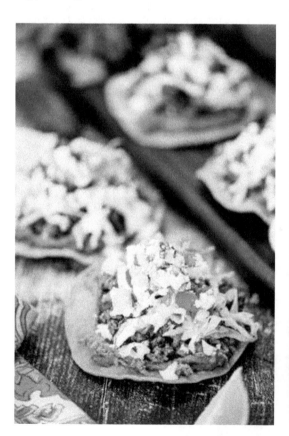

Olive Dip
Prep time: 10 minutes | Cook time: 5 minutes | Serves 4

- 1 clove garlic
- 200 g green pitted olives
- 100 g ground almonds
- 2 tbsp chopped parsley
- 70 ml olive oil
- salt
- Pepper

1. Peel the garlic clove and finely chop it together with the olives in the blender or a tall mixing bowl with the immersion blender.
2. Add the remaining ingredients and mix well.

PER SERVING

Calories: 190 | Protein: 3g | Fat: 19g | Carbohydrates: 2g | Fiber: 3g

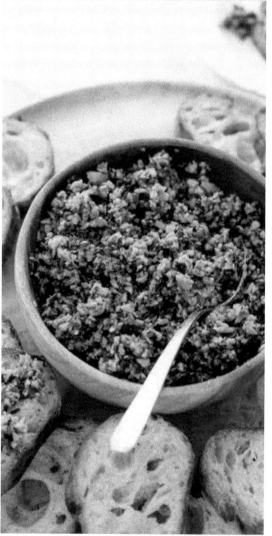

Omelet with Tomatoes

Prep time: 10 minutes | **Cook time:** 15 minutes | **Serves 4**

- 1 shallot
- 100g feta
- 2 sundried tomatoes
- 2 fresh tomatoes
- 3 eggs
- 2 tbsp mineral water
- salt
- pepper
- 2 tbsp canola oil

1. Peel and dice the shallot. Crumble the feta. Cut the sun-dried tomatoes into thin slices. Wash, halve, deseed and finely dice the fresh tomatoes.
2. Whisk the eggs with salt, pepper, and mineral water. Heat the oil in a pan and fry the shallots until golden. Pour in the egg mixture, sprinkle with the feta and tomatoes and leave to set over low heat. Halve the omelet and arrange it on two plates.

PER SERVING

Calories: 315 | Protein: 18g | Fat: 21g | Carbohydrates: 6g

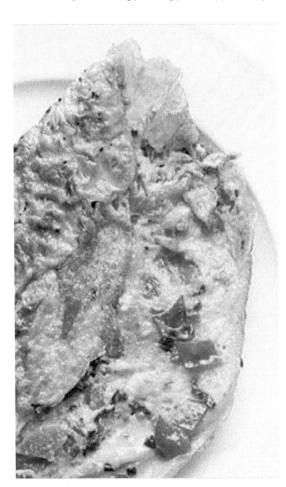

Parmesan Meatballs with Tomato Sauce

Prep time: 10 minutes | **Cook time:** 15 minutes | **Serves 4**

- 200 g minced beef
- 1 egg
- 1 egg yolk
- 1 tbsp chopped parsley
- 100g Parmesan
- 1 clove of garlic
- salt
- pepper
- 1 1/2 tbsp frying oil, e.g. B. Refined olive oil
- 1 small onion
- 400 g (canned) tomatoes
- 1 tsp tomato paste
- 1 tsp dried oregano
- possibly chili powder
- 3 basil leaves

1. Put the minced meat, egg, egg yolk, parsley, and grated Parmesan in a bowl and knead well. Peel the garlic, chop finely and mix in—season with salt and pepper and shape into balls.
2. Heat 1 tbsp oil in a pan, fry the balls briefly and remove.
3. Peel the onions and cut them into fine rings, sauté in the frying fat. Add the tomato pieces with salt, pepper, tomato paste, oregano, and possibly chili powder. Simmer for 5 minutes. Meanwhile, wash the basil, pat dry, and cut into strips. Add the meatballs and basil to the sauce and cook for another 5-7 minutes.

PER SERVING

Calories: 520 | Protein: 48g | Fat: 32g | Carbohydrates: 5g | Fiber: 3g

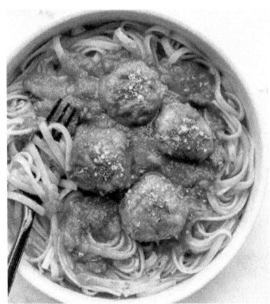

Quark Bowl with Psyllium

Prep time: 10 minutes | Cook time: 15 minutes | Serves 4

- 80g fresh or frozen blueberries
- alternatively: apple or other berries
- 100g lowfat quark
- 30ml milk
- alternatively: unsweetened plant drink
- 1tsp linseed oil
- 1tbsp buckwheat flakes
- 1tbsp Flea Seed Shells

1. Wash fresh berries; place frozen berries in a breakfast bowl to thaw.
2. Mix the quark with milk or plant drink until smooth.
3. Add linseed oil, flakes, and flea seeds.
4. Mix everything and let it soak briefly.

PER SERVING

Calories: 185 | Fat: 7g | Carbohydrates: 13g | Protein: 16g | Fiber: 9g | BE 1

Cottage Cheese Breakfast with Mango

Prep time: 10 minutes | Cook time: 15 minutes | Serves 4

- 0.5 Mango
- 250 g low-fat quark
- 3THE hafer drink
- 1HE linseed
- 1TL Flohsamen
- 1HE sunflower seeds
- 1HE linseed oil

1. Peel the mango and remove the flesh from the pit.
2. Place all the other ingredients in a mixing bowl and blend until smooth.

PER SERVING

Calories: 431 | Fat: 18g | Carbohydrates: 25g | Protein: 40g | Fiber: 8g | BE 2.1

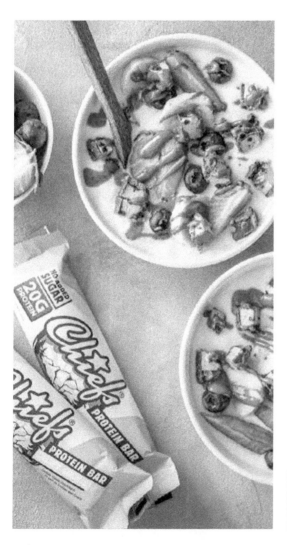
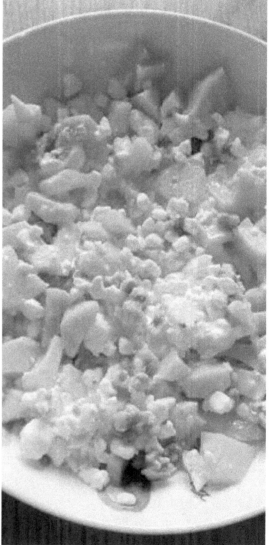

Rye bun

Prep time: 10 minutes | Cook time: 55 minutes | Serves 4

- 200 g rye flour type 1370
- 50 g rye grist type 1800
- 200ml of water
- 1 cube of yeast
- 25 g butter at room temperature
- 1tsp sea salt

1. Put the rye flour and rye meal in a bowl and make a well in the middle. Crumble the yeast into a little lukewarm water and stir well. Pour the dissolved yeast into the well and let this pre-dough rise for about 20 minutes.
2. Then add the remaining ingredients and knead everything together well. The consistency of the dough is correct if it still slightly sticks to your hands. Cover and let rise for at least 40 minutes.
3. If necessary, knead again, form long rolls with slightly damp hands and cut them once or twice on the top. Let rise for about 20-30 minutes and bake for 30-40 minutes at 200 degrees.

PER SERVING

Calories: 176 | Protein: 6g | Fat: 4g | Carbohydrates: 29g | Fiber: 5g

Beetroot Salad with Wholemeal Bread

Prep time: 10 minutes | Cook time: 15 minutes | Serves 1

- 1 bulb of cooked beetroot
- 1/2 apple
- 1 carrot
- 1 tbsp lemon juice
- 30 ml vegetable broth
- 1 tsp horseradish
- 1/4 bunch of fresh herbs, egg, chives, or parsley
- freshly ground pepper
- 1 slice of wholemeal bread

1. Thinly slice the beets and place them in a bowl. Wash, clean, and grate the apple and carrot. Mix everything.
2. Whisk together the lemon juice, broth, and horseradish for the dressing, mix the vegetables, and leave to infuse. Wash the herbs, shake dry, chop finely, and mix with pepper loosely.
3. Serve the raw vegetable salad with wholemeal bread.

PER SERVING

Calories: 228 | Protein: 7g | Fat: 2g | Carbohydrates: 45g | Fiber: 12g

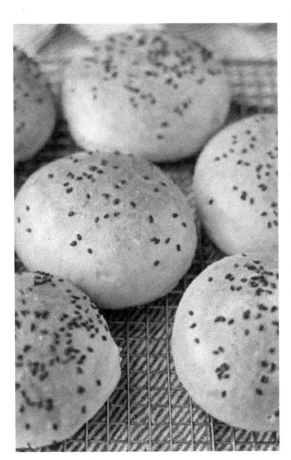
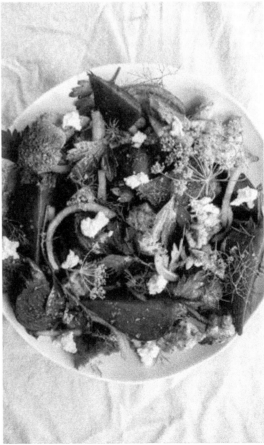

Homemade Kefir

Prep time: 10 minutes | **Cook time:** 15 minutes | **Serves 4**

- Ingredients for 1 glass:
- 1tbsp kefir mushroom
- 500 ml (3.5% fat) UHT milk

1. Pour the room-temperature milk into a screw-top glass with a wide opening. Use a wooden or plastic spoon to slide the kefir fungus into the milk and close tightly. Leave the culture at room temperature 16-23 degrees for 36 to a maximum of 48 hours.
2. After one and a half to two days, pour the finished kefir through a fine-mesh plastic sieve and enjoy either pure or pureed fruit.

PER SERVING

Calories: 128 | Carbohydrates: 7g | Fat: 7g | Protein: 7g | Fiber: 0g | BE 0.6

Smoothie with Strawberries and Barley Grass

Prep time: 10 minutes | **Cook time:** 15 minutes | **Serves 2**

- 1banana
- 100 grams of strawberries
- Optional: 50 g lettuce
- 1-3 tsp barley grass powder
- 1tbsp peeled hemp seeds
- 150ml of water

1. Peel and slice the banana. Next, wash the strawberries, remove the stems and pat dry. Also, wash and chop the lettuce (e.g., endives, lamb's lettuce, rocket, radicchio, oak leaf lettuce).
2. Put everything in a blender with hemp seeds, barley grass powder, water, and puree into a smoothie. If you don't have a blender, just use a blender. Pour into a tall glass and enjoy.

PER SERVING

Calories: 183 | Fat: 5g | Carbohydrates: 27g | Protein: 7g | Fiber: 9g | BE 2.2

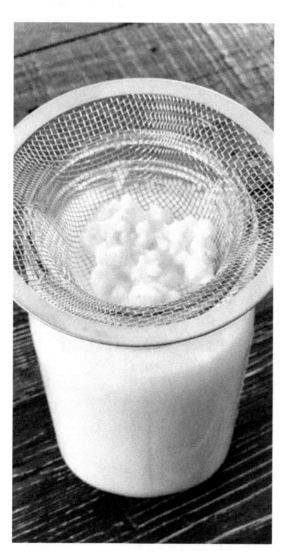
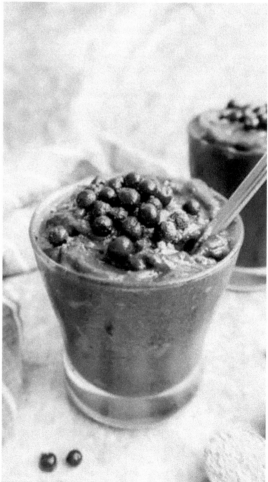

Smoothie with Mango, Grapefruit and Parsley

Prep time: 10 minutes | Cook time: 15 minutes | Serves 4

- 20 grams of parsley
- 1 Orange
- 1 Grapefruit
- 1 Mango
- 100ml of water
- 1tsp linseed oil
- 1tsp wheat germ oil

1. Wash the parsley well and peel the fruit.
2. Remove the flesh from the mango and roughly chop the fruit.
3. Finely puree all the ingredients together in a blender or hand blender.

PER SERVING

Calories: 240 | Protein: 5g | Fat: 6g | Carbohydrates: 36g | Fiber: 5g

Smoothie with Spinach and Strawberries

Prep time: 10 minutes | Cook time: 5 minutes | Serves 4

- 150ml of water
- 250g spinach
- 5 large strawberries
- 1 pear
- 1tbsp linseed oil
- 1tbsp wheat germ oil

1. Wash and trim strawberries. Wash, quarter and core the pear. Wash the fresh spinach. Frozen spinach works just as well - roughly chop if necessary.
2. Finely puree all ingredients together in a blender or with a hand blender.

PER SERVING

Calories: 130 | Protein: 4g | Fat: 7g | Carbohydrates: 11g | Fiber: 5g

Asparagus salad with chicken

Prep time: 10 minutes | Cook time: 15 minutes | Serves 4

- 1tbsp pumpkin seeds
- 200g asparagus
- 200g zucchini
- 3 spring onions
- 0.5 organic lemon
- 240g chicken breast fillet
- salt
- from the mill: pepper
- 2tbsp olive oil
- 2tsp butter
- 100ml gluten free vegetable broth
- 1tsp liquid honey
- 2tbsp Creme fraiche Cheese

1. Roast the pumpkin seeds in a pan without fat until light, remove and allow to cool. Wash and peel the asparagus, cut off the ends, cut the stalks into slices at an angle. Wash and dice zucchini. Clean and wash the spring onions and cut crosswise into pieces about 4 cm long.
2. Wash the lemon in hot water, finely grate the zest and squeeze out the juice (about 0.5 tablespoons per portion). Wash the meat, pat dry, season with lemon zest, salt, and pepper—Fry in half the oil in a grill pan over medium-high heat for about 15 minutes.
3. Meanwhile, heat the remaining oil and butter in another pan fry the asparagus for 8-10 minutes while turning. Add zucchini cubes and spring onions and sauté for about 3 minutes. Add the broth, honey, and crème fraîche and simmer, with the lid on, over medium heat for about 5 minutes until al dente. Season with salt, pepper, and lemon juice.
4. Divide the cooked chicken into bite-sized pieces, fold it into the fried vegetables, and sprinkle with the pumpkin seeds. Serve warm or cold.

PER SERVING

Calories: 420 | Carbohydrates: 13g | Protein: 36g | Fat: 24g | Fiber: 4g | BE 1

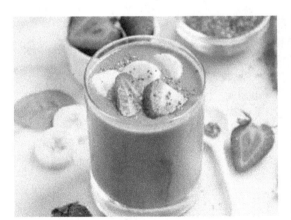
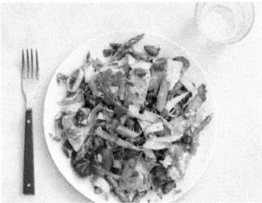

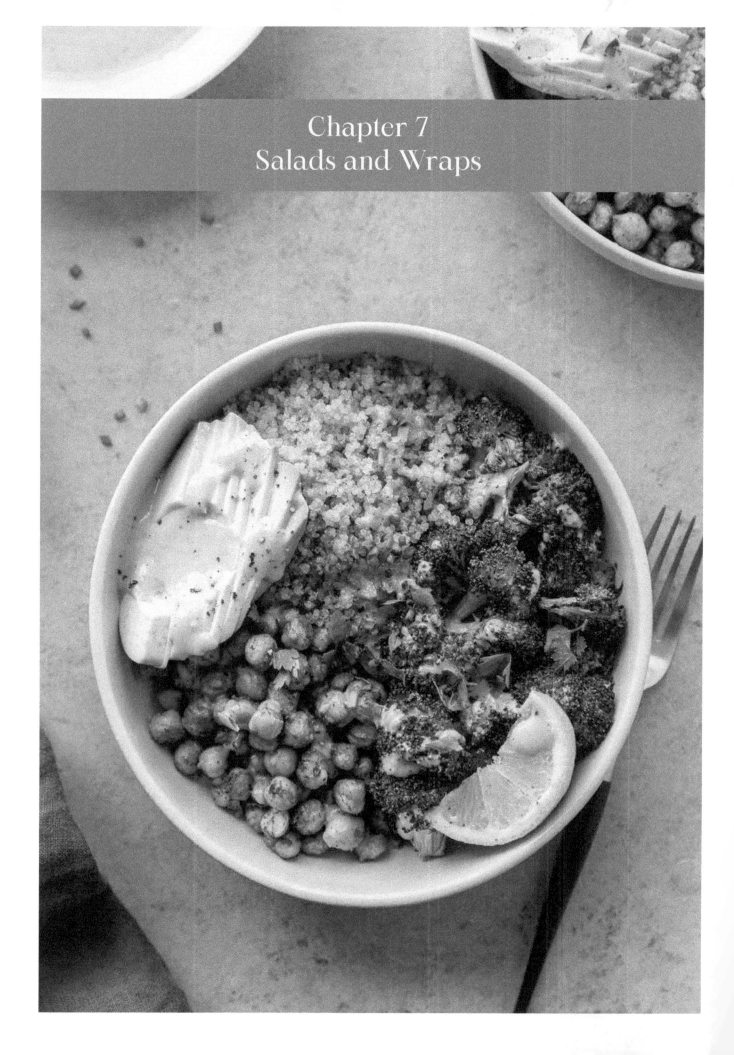

Chapter 7
Salads and Wraps

Quinoa & Chickpea Grain Bowl

Prep time: 5 minutes | Cook time: 15 minutes | Serves 1

- ⅓ cup of chickpeas (canned), rinsed then drained
- 1 cup of cooked quinoa
- ½ cup of cucumber slices
- ¼ diced avocado
- ½ cup of cherry tomatoes, halved
- 3 tbsp. of hummus
- 1 tbsp. of lemon juice
- 1 tbsp. of roasted red pepper, finely chopped
- 1 tbsp. of water, plus some more if desired
- Pinch of salt
- 1 tsp. of fresh parsley, chopped (Optional)
- Pinch of pepper, ground

1. In a large mixing bowl, combine the quinoa, cucumbers, chickpeas, tomatoes, and avocado.
2. In a mixing bowl, combine the hummus, lemon juice, roasted red pepper, and water. To get the appropriate dressing consistency, add additional water. Stir in the parsley, salt, and pepper to mix. Serve with a Buddha dish on the side.

PER SERVING

Calories: 220 | Fat: 16.6g | Carbohydrates: 75g | Protein: 17.9g

Green Salad with Hummus & Pita Bread

Prep time: 5 minutes | Cook time: 10 minutes | Serves 1

- ½ cup of sliced cucumber
- 2 cups of mixed salad greens
- 2 tbsp. of grated carrot
- 1 and ½ tsp. of balsamic vinegar
- 1 and ½ tsp. of extra-virgin olive oil
- Pinch of salt
- 1 pita bread, whole-wheat (6 and 1/2-inch), toasted
- Pinch of pepper, ground
- ¼ cup of hummus

1. On a big platter, arrange the greens, cucumber, and carrot.
2. Drizzle with olive oil and balsamic vinegar.
3. Season to taste with salt and black pepper.
4. Serve with hummus and pita on the side.

PER SERVING

Calories: 374 | Fat: 14.5g | Carbohydrates: 52.6g | Protein: 13.5g

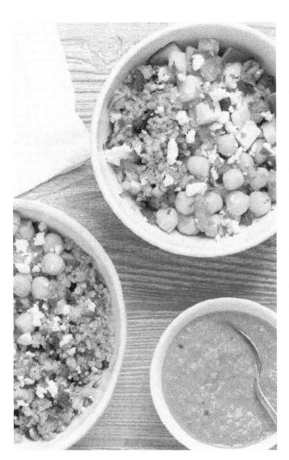
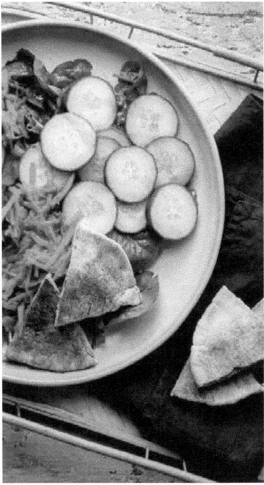

Green Salad with Beets & Edamame

Prep time: 5 minutes | Cook time: 15 minutes | Serves 1

- 1 cup of edamame (shelled), thawed
- 2 cups of mixed salad greens
- ½ raw peeled beet (medium), shredded (almost 1/2 cup)
- 1 tbsp. of fresh cilantro, chopped
- 1 tbsp. of plus 1 and 1/2 tsp. of red-wine vinegar
- Freshly ground black pepper to taste
- 2 tsp. of extra-virgin olive oil

1. On a big platter, arrange the greens, edamame, and beet.
2. In a small bowl, combine the vinegar, oil, cilantro, salt, and pepper.
3. Drizzle the dressing over salad and serve.

PER SERVING

Calories: 325 | Fat: 15.7g | Carbohydrates: 25.5g | Protein: 18.5g

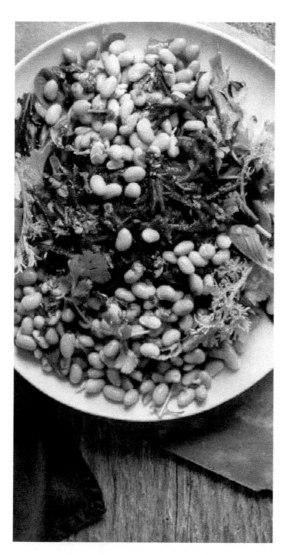

Classic Mason jar Cobb Salad

Prep time: 5 minutes | Cook time: 20 minutes | Serves 1

- 2 tbsp. of chopped cucumber
- 2 tbsp. of Blue Cheese Creamy Dressing
- 2 tbsp. of chopped tomato
- 1 ounce of chopped deli ham (low or reduced sodium)
- 2 tbsp. of diced red onion
- 1 ounce of chopped deli turkey (low or reduced sodium)
- 1 slice of crisply bacon (cooked), crumbled
- 1 egg (hard-boiled), diced
- ½ cubed avocado
- 1 tbsp. of crumbled blue cheese
- 1 and ½ cups of romaine lettuce, chopped
- 1 tsp. of lime juice

1. Fill a mason jar (quart-size) halfway with blue cheese dressing. Tomato, Cucumber, and onion go on top. Ham, egg, turkey, and bacon are layered on top of each other. In a small dish, gently combine the avocado with the lime juice, then add to container.
2. Blue cheese should be sprinkled on top of the salad. Fill the jar with the lettuce to fill the empty space. Refrigerate the jar with the lid on.
3. Shake the salad out of the container onto a dish when ready to serve.

PER SERVING

Calories: 422 | Fat: 28.5g | Carbohydrates: 19.5g | Protein: 24.9g

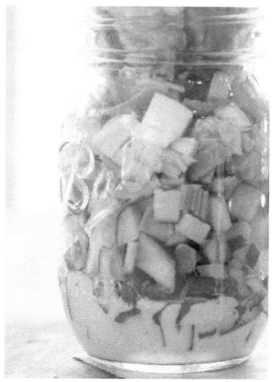

Green Salad with Chickpeas

Prep time: 5 minutes | Cook time: 15 minutes | Serves 2

- 1 and ½ cups of buttermilk
- 1 peeled avocado, pitted
- ¼ cup of fresh herbs (chopped), like sorrel, tarragon, parsley mint and/or cilantro
- ½ tsp. of salt
- 2 tbsp. of rice vinegar
- 1 cup of sliced cucumber
- 3 cups of romaine lettuce, chopped
- 1 can of chickpeas (15 ounce), rinsed
- 6 halved cherry tomatoes, if desired
- ¼ cup of diced Swiss cheese (low-fat)

1. To make the dressing, follow these steps: In a blender, combine the avocado, herbs, buttermilk, vinegar, and salt. Puree until completely smooth.
2. To make a salad, follow these steps: Toss the lettuce and cucumber with 1/4 cup of dressing in a mixing bowl. Chickpeas, cheese, and tomatoes go on top. (Keep the excess dressing refrigerated for max. 3 days.)

PER SERVING

Calories: 304 | Fat: 7.5g | Carbohydrates: 39.8g | Protein: 21.7g

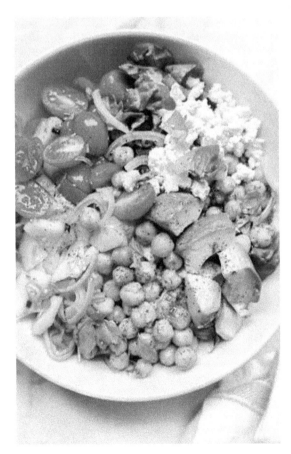

Stuffed Avocados Chicken Salad

Prep time: 5 minutes | Cook time: 50 minutes | Serves 4

- ⅓ cup of plain Greek yogurt (low-fat)
- 1 pound of skinless, boneless chicken breast
- ¼ cup of mayonnaise
- ¾ tsp. of salt
- 1 tbsp. of fresh tarragon, chopped
- ½ tsp. of ground pepper
- 1 cup of red grapes (seedless), halved (Optional)
- 1 cup of diced celery
- ¼ cup of toasted chopped pecans
- 2 firm avocados (ripe), halved & pitted

1. In a large saucepan, place enough water and the chicken to cover it. Over medium heat, bring to a simmer. Reduce heat to a low simmer, cover, and cook for 12 to 15 minutes, or until an instant-read thermometer reads 165 degrees F. Place on a chopping board to cool. Allow to cool completely before chopping or shredding. Refrigerate for 30 minutes or until completely cool.
2. In a large mixing bowl, combine the yogurt, mayonnaise, tarragon, salt, and pepper. Stir in the chilled chicken, grapes, celery (if using), and pecans.
3. To serve, spoon roughly 1/2 cup of chicken salad into each avocado half. (Keep the leftover chicken salad refrigerated for max. 3 days.)

PER SERVING

Calories: 308 | Fat: 24g | Carbohydrates: 10g | Protein: 16.1g

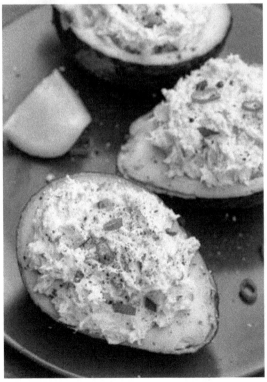

Apple & Chicken Kale Wraps

Prep time: 5 minutes | Cook time: 10 minutes | Serves 1

- 1 tsp. of Dijon mustard
- 1 tbsp. of mayonnaise
- 3 lacinato kale leaves (medium)
- 6 red onion slices, thin
- 3 ounces of cooked chicken breast, thinly sliced
- 1 apple (firm), cut in 9 slices

1. In a small bowl, combine mayonnaise and mustard.
2. Apply to kale leaves.
3. 1 ounce of chicken, 2 onion slices, and 3 apple slices per leaf Make a wrap out of each leaf.
4. If desired, cut in half.

PER SERVING

Calories: 370 | Fat: 13.7g | Carbohydrates: 34.1g | Protein: 29.3g

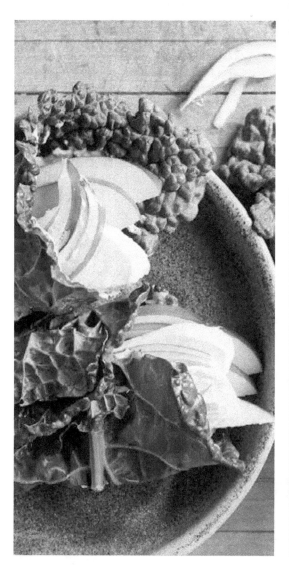

Greek Edamame Salad

Prep time: 5 minutes | Cook time: 20 minutes | Serves 4

- 3 tbsp. of extra-virgin olive oil
- ¼ cup of red-wine vinegar
- ¼ tsp. of salt
- 8 cups of romaine, chopped (about two romaine hearts)
- ¼ tsp. of ground pepper
- 16 ounces of shelled edamame, frozen (about three cups), thawed
- ½ sliced European cucumber
- 1 cup of halved grape or cherry tomatoes
- ½ cup of crumbled feta cheese
- ¼ cup of Kalamata olives, sliced
- ¼ cup of slivered fresh basil
- ¼ cup of slivered red onion

1. In a large mixing bowl, combine the vinegar, oil, salt, and pepper.
2. Toss in the romaine, tomatoes, edamame, cucumber, basil, feta, olives, and onion.

PER SERVING

Calories: 344 | Fat: 23.3g | Carbohydrates: 19.9g | Protein: 17.1g

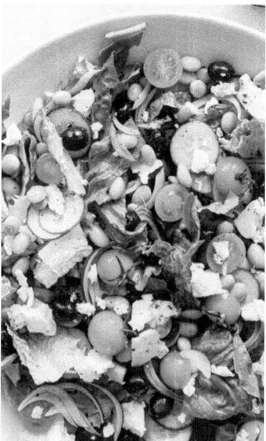

Spring Roll Salad

Prep time: 5 minutes | Cook time: 10 minutes | Serves 1

- 1 and ½ tsp. of sesame oil
- 1 tbsp. of natural peanut butter
- 1 and ½ tsp. of rice vinegar
- 1 tsp. of soy sauce or tamari
- 1 tsp. of maple syrup
- 1 tsp. of water
- Pinch of red pepper, crushed (optional)
- ½ tsp. of minced garlic
- 3 cups of butter lettuce or torn Boston
- ½ cup of cooked brown rice
- 3 ounces of cooked shrimp
- ¼ cup of chopped red cabbage
- ¼ cup of julienned carrots
- ¼ cup of julienned bell pepper
- ¼ cup of julienned cucumber
- sesame seeds and Fresh mint for garnish
- ¼ cup of avocado

1. In a small bowl, whisk together peanut butter, rice vinegar, oil, maple syrup, soy sauce (or tamari), water, garlic, and red pepper (if using).
2. In a mixing bowl, combine the lettuce, rice, shrimp, cabbage, carrot, bell pepper, cucumber, and avocado. Toss in the dressing to mix. If desired, garnish with sesame and mint seeds.

PER SERVING

Calories: 523 | Fat: 24.9g | Carbohydrates: 44.5g | Protein: 31g

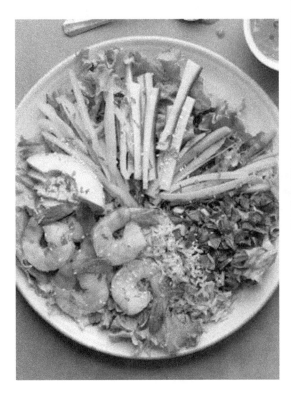

Turkey Kale Wraps

Prep time: 5 minutes | Cook time: 10 minutes | Serves 1

- 1 tsp. of Dijon mustard
- 1 tbsp. of cranberry sauce
- 3 lacinato kale leaves (medium)
- 6 red onion, in thin slices
- 3 slices of deli turkey (almost about 3 ounces)
- 1 firm pear (ripe), cut in 9 slices

1. In a small bowl, combine the cranberry sauce and mustard.
2. Apply to kale leaves.
3. Add a piece of turkey, two slices of red onion, and three slices of pear to each leaf.
4. Make a wrap out of each leaf. If desired, cut each of the wraps in half.

PER SERVING

Calories: 293 | Fat: 2.1g | Carbohydrates: 42.6g | Protein: 27.8g

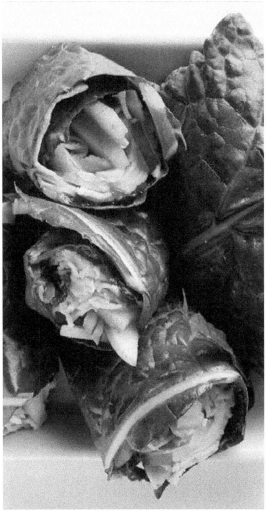

Shrimp & Avocado Chopped Salad

Prep time: 5 minutes | Cook time: 50 minutes | Serves 4

- 3 tbsp. of extra-virgin olive oil or grape-seed oil
- 5 tbsp. of sour cream (reduced-fat)
- 3 tbsp. of cider vinegar
- 1 tbsp. of chopped fresh dill
- 2 tbsp. of chopped fresh cilantro
- 1 tbsp. of minced shallot
- ¾ tsp. of dry mustard
- 2 cloves of garlic, minced
- ¼ tsp. of kosher salt
- 2 tsp. of extra-virgin olive oil
- 1 pound of raw shrimp (21 to 25 per pound), peeled, then deveined
- 2 tsp. of lime zest, finely grated
- ¼ tsp. of pepper (freshly ground), plus some more to taste
- ¼ tsp. of kosher salt
- 2 ears of corn, husked
- ¾ cup of red cabbage, finely chopped
- 4 cups of chopped romaine lettuce
- ¾ cup of red bell pepper, diced
- ½ cup of cherry tomatoes, chopped
- ½ cup of diced red onion
- ½ halved fennel bulb, thinly sliced
- 2 slices of crispy bacon (cooked), diced
- 1 diced avocado

1. To make the dressing, follow these steps: In a blender or food processor, puree dressing ingredients until smooth.
2. Preheat the grill to the medium or place a grill pan on medium heat to prepare the shrimp and salad.
3. Toss shrimp with the 2 tsp. oil, salt, lime zest, and 1/4 tsp. pepper.
4. Grill corn for 6 to 10 minutes, stirring regularly, until slightly browned. Grill the shrimp for 3 to 5 minutes, rotating once, until cooked through. Toss the corn and shrimp together on a chopping board. Remove the corn kernels from the cob. Cut the shrimp into small pieces.
5. In a large mixing bowl, combine cabbage, lettuce, bell pepper, tomatoes, onion, avocado, fennel, and bacon. Toss in the shrimp, corn, and dressing to combine. Season with salt and black pepper.

PER SERVING

Calories: 398 | Fat: 25g | Carbohydrates: 21.5g | Protein: 25.8g

Green Goddess Chicken Salad

Prep time: 5 minutes | Cook time: 15 minutes | Serves 1

- 1 and ½ cups of buttermilk
- 1 peeled avocado, pitted
- ¼ cup of fresh herbs, chopped (such as sorrel, tarragon, parsley, mint, and/or cilantro)
- ½ tsp. of salt
- 2 tbsp. of rice vinegar
- 1 cup of sliced cucumber
- 3 cups of chopped romaine lettuce
- 3 ounces of diced (or sliced) cooked skinless, boneless chicken breast
- 6 halved cherry tomatoes, if desired
- ½ cup of diced Swiss cheese, low-fat (2 ounces)

1. To make the dressing, purée the avocado with the buttermilk, herbs, vinegar, and salt in a blender until smooth. (This recipe yields approximately 1 and 3/4 cup dressing.)
2. To make a salad, follow these steps: Toss the lettuce and cucumber with 1 tbsp. of the dressing in a mixing bowl. Chicken, cheese, and tomatoes go on top. (Keep the excess dressing refrigerated for max. 3 days.)

PER SERVING

Calories: 296 | Fat: 7.4g | Carbohydrates: 14.5g | Protein: 43g

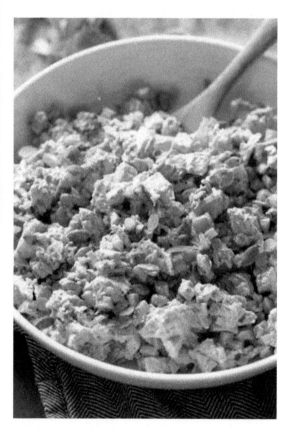

Chicken Club Wraps

Prep time: 5 minutes | **Cook time:** 30 minutes | **Serves 4**

- ½ tsp. of pepper (freshly ground), divided
- 1 pound of skinless, boneless chicken breast, trimmed
- 3 tbsp. of plain Greek yogurt (nonfat)
- 3 tbsp. of minced onion
- 3 tbsp. of cider vinegar
- 2 tbsp. of extra-virgin olive oil
- 1 tomato (medium), chopped
- ⅛ tsp. of salt
- 1 chopped avocado
- 8 leaves of green or red leaf lettuce (large)
- 3 strips of cooked bacon, crumbled
- 4 flour tortillas (10-inch), whole-wheat

1. Preheat the grill to medium to high temperature.
2. Put 1/4 tsp. pepper on both sides of the chicken Grease the grill rack. Grill the chicken for 15 to 18 minutes, rotating once or twice, till an instant-read thermometer put into the thickest section registers 165°F. Allow it cool for approximately 5 minutes on a clean chopping board.
3. In a large mixing bowl, whisk together the yogurt, vinegar, onion, oil, salt, and the other 1/4 tsp. pepper. Chop your chicken in bite-size pieces and put with the tomato, avocado, and bacon in a mixing bowl; toss to blend.
4. Place two lettuce leaves on each of the tortilla and top it with chicken salad to make the wraps (about 1 cup each). Like a tortilla, roll it up. If preferred, serve sliced in half.

PER SERVING

Calories: 526 | Fat: 25.6g | Carbohydrates: 39g | Protein: 33.6g

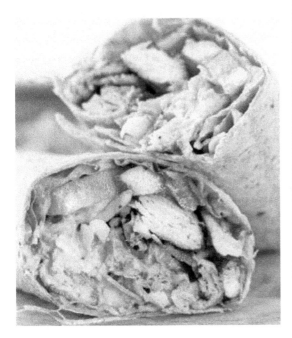

Mediterranean Antipasto Tuna Salad

Prep time: 5 minutes | **Cook time:** 25 minutes | **Serves 4**

- 2 cans of chunk light tuna, water-packed (5-6 ounce), drained & flaked
- 1 can of beans (15-19 ounce), like kidney beans, black-eyed peas or chickpeas, rinsed
- 1 red bell pepper (large), finely diced
- ½ cup of fresh parsley (chopped), divided
- ½ cup of red onion, finely chopped
- 4 tsp. of capers, rinsed
- ½ cup of lemon juice, divided
- 1 and ½ tsp. of fresh rosemary, finely chopped
- 4 tbsp. of olive oil, divided
- ¼ tsp. of salt
- Freshly ground black pepper, to taste
- 8 cups of mixed salad greens

1. In a medium mixing bowl, combine the beans, bell pepper, tuna, onion, capers, parsley, 1/4 cup lemon juice, rosemary, and 2 tbsp. oil.
2. Season with salt and pepper. In a large mixing bowl, combine the other 1/4 cup of lemon juice, 2 tbsp. oil, and salt. Toss in the salad greens to coat. Distribute the greens amongst four plates. Toss the tuna salad on top of each serving.

PER SERVING

Calories: 306 | Fat: 15.9g | Carbohydrates: 28.5g | Protein: 14.8g

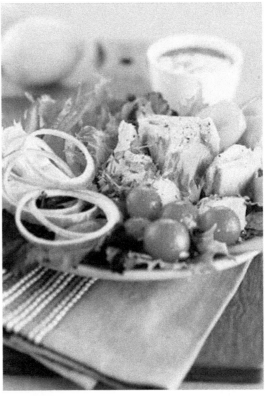

The Cobb Salad

Prep time: 5 minutes | Cook time: 40 minutes | Serves 4

- 2 tbsp. of finely minced shallot
- 3 tbsp. of white-wine vinegar
- 1 tbsp. of Dijon mustard
- ¼ tsp. of salt
- 1 tsp. of freshly ground pepper
- 3 tbsp. of extra-virgin olive oil
- 8 ounces of shredded chicken breast, cooked (about 1 breast half, large)
- 10 cups of mixed salad greens
- 2 hard-boiled eggs (large), peeled then chopped
- 1 cucumber (large), seeded & sliced
- 2 tomatoes (medium), diced
- 1 diced avocado
- 1/2 cup of blue cheese (crumbled), (optional)
- 2 slices of cooked bacon, crumbled

1. In a small mixing bowl, combine the vinegar, shallot, mustard, pepper, and salt. Whisk in the oil until it's all blended. In a large mixing basin, combine the salad greens. Toss in half of dressing to coat.
2. Distribute the greens amongst four plates. On top of the lettuce, layer equal amounts of chicken, tomatoes, egg, cucumber, bacon, avocado, and blue cheese (if using). Drizzle the remaining dressing over the salads.

PER SERVING

Calories: 379 | Fat: 24.8g | Carbohydrates: 15g | Protein: 26.6g

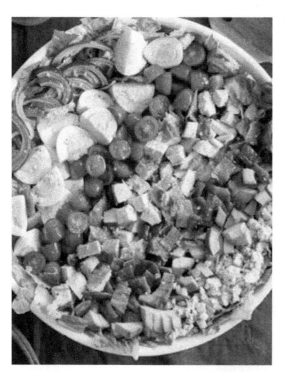

Power Salad

Prep time: 5 minutes | Cook time: 10 minutes | Serves 1

- ¾ cup of cottage cheese (nonfat)
- 1 shallot (small), peeled
- ¼ cup of reduced-fat mayonnaise
- 2 tbsp. of white-wine vinegar
- 2 tbsp. of buttermilk powder
- ¼ cup of nonfat milk
- ¼ tsp. of salt
- 1 tbsp. of chopped dill
- ¼ tsp. of freshly ground pepper
- 1 cup of shredded carrots
- 6 cups of mixed salad greens
- 2 tbsp. of red onion, chopped
- 4 slices (3 ounces) of turkey breast (roast), cut up
- 10 cherry tomatoes
- 2 slices (2 ounces) of Swiss cheese (reduced-fat), cut up

1. To make the dressing, put the shallot via the feed tube to the food processor and pulse until finely chopped. Combine the mayonnaise, cottage cheese, buttermilk powder, and vinegar in a mixing bowl. Process for 3 minutes, scraping down the edges as needed, until smooth. While processor is running, pour in the milk. Scrape down the sides of the bowl, then add the dill, salt, and black pepper and process until smooth. (This recipe yields 1 1/4 cup.)
2. To make a salad, follow these steps: In a large mixing bowl, toss the greens, onion, carrots, and 1/4 cup dressing until well combined. Divide the mixture between two plates. Toss the salad with tomatoes, turkey, and cheese.

PER SERVING

Calories: 187 | Fat: 3.2g | Carbohydrates: 21.5g | Protein: 19.5g

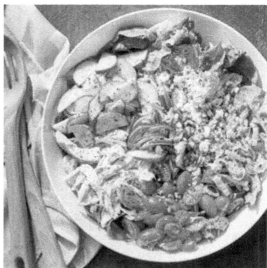

Healthy Shrimp Artichoke Green Salad

Prep time: 5 minutes | Cook time: 30 minutes | Serves 4

- ¾ cup of nonfat buttermilk
- ½ peeled avocado, pitted
- 2 tbsp. of fresh herbs (chopped), such as sorrel, tarragon and/or chives
- 1 tsp. of minced anchovy fillet, or anchovy paste
- 2 tsp. of white-wine vinegar, or tarragon vinegar
- 8 cups of green leaf lettuce, bite-size pieces
- ½ sliced cucumber
- 12 ounces of peeled shrimp, deveined and cooked (21-25 each pound)
- 1 cup of grape or cherry tomatoes
- 1 cup of canned artichoke hearts (rinsed), chopped
- 1 cup of chickpeas (canned), rinsed
- ½ cup of chopped celery

1. In a blender, puree the avocado, buttermilk, herbs, vinegar, and anchovy until smooth.
2. Place lettuce on four plates. Shrimp, tomatoes, cucumber, artichoke hearts, chickpeas, and celery are served on top. Dress the salads with the dressing.

PER SERVING

Calories: 262 | Fat: 6.4g | Carbohydrates: 31.1g | Protein: 22g

Chicken Milanese and Arugula Salad

Prep time: 5 minutes | Cook time: 25 minutes | Serves 4

- 4 skinless, boneless chicken breasts (6-ounce)
- 3 tbsp. of olive oil, plus some more for a grill
- ½ tsp. of ground coriander
- 3 tbsp. of fresh lemon juice
- Some kosher salt and pepper
- 5 ounces (about 6 cups) of baby arugula
- ½ red onion (small), sliced
- 4 sliced radishes

1. Preheat the grill to high heat. Wipe the grill grate using a wire brush once it's hot. Oil grill grate just before you start cooking.
2. Cut each chicken breast in half horizontally (don't cut it all the way through); split and pound to a thickness of 12 inches.
3. Coriander, 1/2 tsp. salt, and 1/4 tsp. Pepper is used to seasoning the chicken. 2 to 3 minutes on each side on the grill until cooked through.
4. In a large mixing bowl, combine the lemon juice, oil, 1/2 teaspoon salt, and 1/4 teaspoon pepper. Toss in the radishes, arugula, and onion until everything is well combined. Pour the sauce over the chicken.

PER SERVING

Calories: 289 | Fat: 14g | Carbohydrates: 3g | Protein: 35g

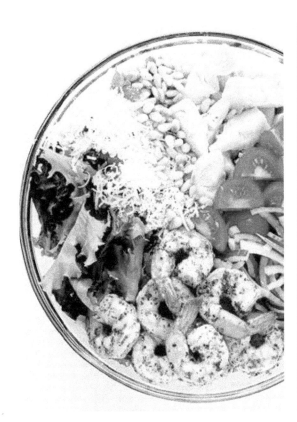

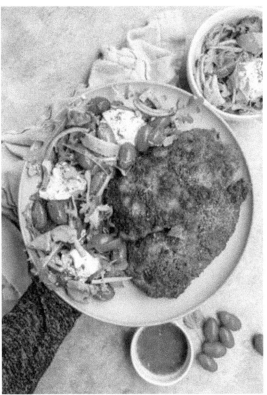

Crunchy Lettuce Chicken Wraps

Prep time: 5 minutes | Cook time: 30 minutes | Serves 4

- ¼ cup of lime juice (fresh), from 3 limes
- Canola or Vegetable oil, for grill grates
- ¼ cup of fish sauce
- 2 tbsp. of Sriracha or Sambal Oelek (chili paste, ground fresh)
- 3 cloves of garlic, grated (2 tsp.)
- 1 tbsp. of granulated sugar
- 4 ounces of rice vermicelli noodles
- 2 pounds of skinless, boneless chicken thighs
- 1 head of butter lettuce or green leaf lettuce, leaves separated
- Some shaved rainbow carrots & cucumber matchsticks to serve

1. Preheat the grill pan or grill to medium to high (450°F-500°F) and brush the grates liberally with oil. On the stove, bring a big pot of water to boil.
2. In a small bowl, whisk together lime juice, garlic, fish sauce, sugar, Sambal Oelek, and 1/4 cup water until sugar dissolves. 1/3 cup sauce should be transferred to a medium bowl; the remaining sauce should be saved until dishing. Toss the chicken in a medium mixing basin and toss to coat. Allow for a 5-minute rest period.
3. In the meantime, prepare the noodles according to the package directions. Set aside after draining and rinsing under cold water.
4. Place the marinated chicken on the grill and toss away the marinade. Cover and grill chicken for approximately 8 minutes, flipping periodically until lightly browned and cooked through. Place on the cutting board and cut into small pieces. Serve the chicken with noodles, lettuce leaves, the saved dipping sauce, carrots, and cucumber on a bed of lettuce leaves.

PER SERVING

Calories: 407 | Fat: 13g | Carbohydrates: 27g | Protein: 44g

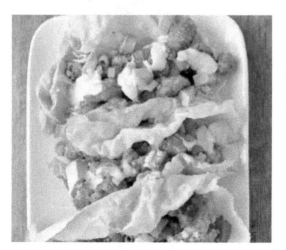

Buttermilk Chicken with Tomato Salad

Prep time: 5 minutes | Cook time: 20 minutes | Serves 4

- ¼ cup of mayonnaise
- ¼ cup of buttermilk
- 1 tbsp. of fresh lemon juice
- Some kosher salt and pepper
- 4 roughly chopped plum tomatoes
- 2 romaine hearts, torn in bite-size pieces
- ½ tbsp. of fresh chives, chopped
- 1 2- to 2 and ½-pound of rotisserie chicken, split up

1. Whisk together the mayonnaise, buttermilk, and lemon juice in a medium mixing bowl. Season with 1/4 teaspoon salt and 1/8 teaspoon pepper, then add the tomatoes. Toss everything together.
2. Serve the lettuce on plates with the chicken on top. Toss the salad with the dressing and tomatoes, then top with the chives.

PER SERVING

Calories: 390 | Fat: 22g | Carbohydrates: 5g | Protein: 42g

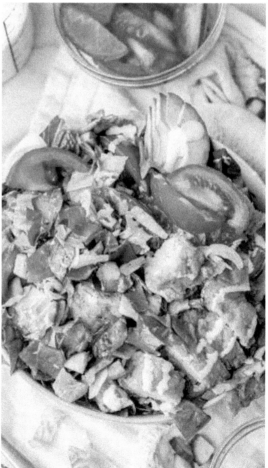

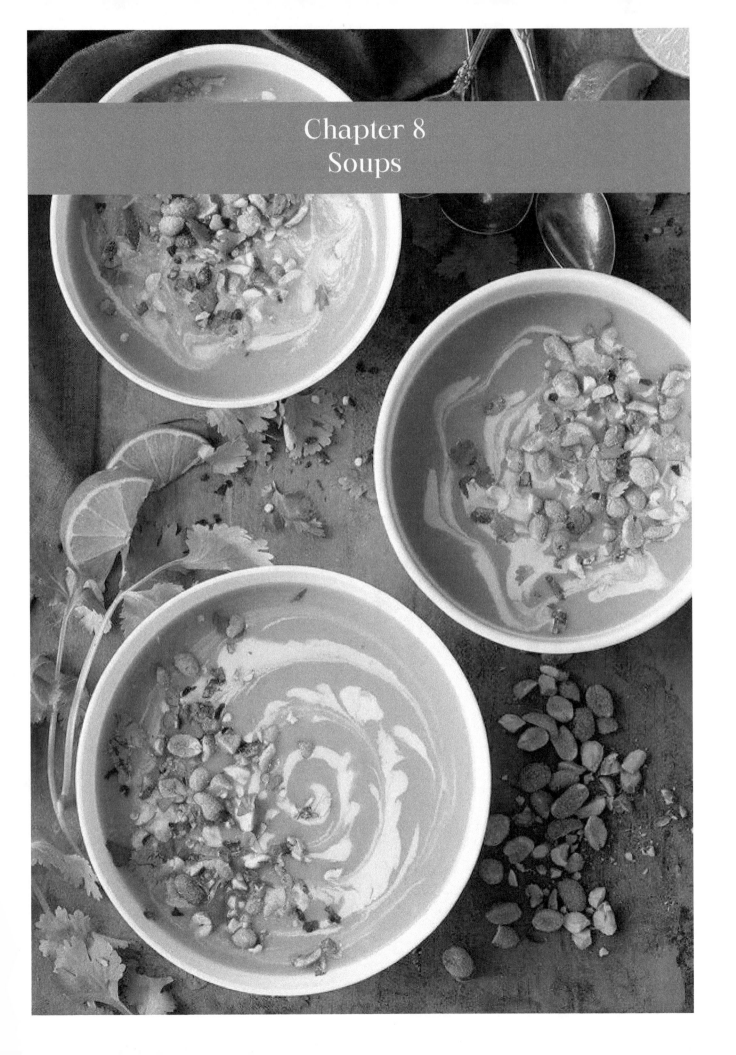

Chapter 8
Soups

Roasted Thai Butternut Squash Soup

Prep time: 5 minutes | Cook time: 1 hour 25 minutes | Serves 4

- 1 sweet potato peeled (large), cut in 1" pieces
- 8 cups of butternut squash, (almost 2.5 pounds), peeled and seeded, cut in 1" pieces
- 2 onion (medium), cut in 1/2" slices
- 1 tsp. of extra virgin olive oil plus 3 tbsp.
- 1/2 tsp. of Thai red curry paste
- 3 cloves of garlic chopped
- 1 inch of ginger peeled and chopped
- 4 cups of vegetable broth (low sodium)
- 1/2 tsp. of salt
- 1/2 cup of light coconut milk
- 1 and 1/2 cups of cooked adzuki beans
- 1/4 tsp. of pepper

1. Preheat the oven up to 400 degrees Fahrenheit. In a large mixing basin, combine the squash, sweet potato, and onion. Drizzle 3 tbsp. of olive oil over the veggies and stir thoroughly.
2. Arrange the veggies in one single layer on a baking sheet coated with parchment paper. Preheat oven to 400°F and bake for 35-40 minutes, or until vegetables are soft.

PER SERVING

Calories: 443 | Fat: 14g | Carbohydrates: 74g | Protein: 11g

Coriander & Carrot soup

Prep time: 5 minutes | Cook time: 35 minutes | Serves 4

- 1 chopped onion
- 1 tbsp. of vegetable oil
- 1 tsp. of ground coriander
- 450g of carrots, peeled & chopped
- 1 chopped potato
- handful of coriander (about half a supermarket packet)
- 1.2 liter of chicken or vegetable stock

1. In a big skillet, heat 1 tablespoon vegetable oil, add one chopped onion, and cook for 5 minutes, or until softened.
2. Cook for 1 minute after adding 1 teaspoon ground coriander & 1 chopped potato.
3. Bring the 450g carrots, peeled and diced, and 1.2L chicken or vegetable stock to a boil, then lower the heat.
4. Cook for 20 minutes, or till the carrots are soft.
5. Blitz with a spoonful of coriander in a food processor till smooth (you may have to do this in 2 batches). Return to the pan, taste, and season with salt if required before reheating to serve.

PER SERVING

Calories: 115 | Fat: 4g | Carbohydrates: 19g | Protein: 3g

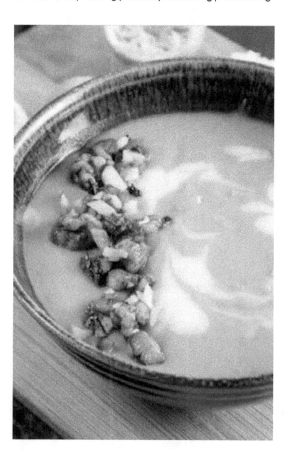
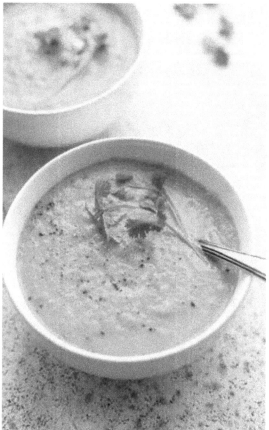

Clear and Healthy Soup

Prep time: 5 minutes | Cook time: 1 hour 45 minutes | Serves 4

- 1 Onion
- 1 pound of Root vegetables
- ½ gallon of Water
- 1 tbsp. of Olive Oil
- 1 Bay Leaf (large) or 2 small
- ¼ tsp. of Nutmeg
- Some Parsley Sprigs
- 7 Juniper Berries
- Lovage, Celery or Allspice Seeds optional
- 10 Peppercorn (Black)
- Salt to taste

1. Remove any contaminants from your root veggies by rinsing them. Slice the onion and cut them into bits.
2. Heat the oil in a big soup pot and sauté the onion pieces.
3. To draw out the flavors, stir in the veggies and sauté for a few minutes.
4. Season with nutmeg, bay leaves, black peppercorns, and juniper berries before adding the water if you have some, season with celery seeds, Lovage, and allspice seeds.
5. Bring the soup to boil, then whisk it briefly. Maintain a constant medium heat setting.
6. Cooking and reducing the soup will allow it to integrate even more flavor over time. This might take anything from 60 to 80 minutes.
7. When it's finished cooking, season it with salt.
8. Using a fine strainer or cheesecloth, strain the soup. The vegetables are used in another meal.
9. Return the strained soup to the heat source. Keep it warm until it's ready to serve.

PER SERVING

Calories: 129 | Fat: 4g | Carbohydrates: 23g | Protein: 2g

Stilton & Broccoli Soup

Prep time: 5 minutes | Cook time: 45 minutes | Serves 4

- 1 finely chopped onion
- 2 tbsp. of rapeseed oil
- 1 stick of celery, sliced
- 1 potato (medium), diced
- 1 sliced leek
- 1 knob of butter
- 1 head of broccoli, roughly chopped
- 1l of homemade or low salt vegetable or chicken stock
- 140g of stilton, or any other crumbled blue cheese

1. In a large saucepan, heat 2 tablespoons rapeseed oil, then add one finely chopped onion. Cook until soft over medium heat. If the onion begins to catch, add a dash of water.
2. 1 celery stick chopped, 1 leek sliced, 1 medium diced potato, and one knob of butter and Cover it with a lid after stirring until melted. Allow for 5 minutes of sweating before removing the cover.
3. 1 liter chicken or vegetable stock, plus any chunky parts of broccoli stem from 1 head of broccoli Cook until all of the veggies are tender, about 10-15 minutes.
4. Cook for another 5 minutes after adding the remainder of the coarsely chopped broccoli.
5. Transfer to the blender and pulse until completely smooth.
6. Allow some lumps to remain after adding 140g crushed stilton. Serve with a pinch of black pepper.

PER SERVING

Calories: 340 | Fat: 21g | Carbohydrates: 13.8g | Protein: 24.3g

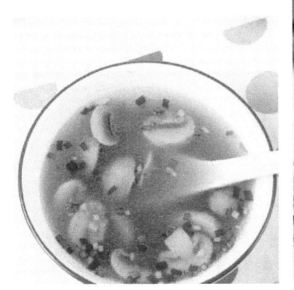

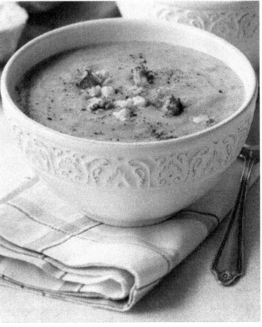

Celery soup

Prep time: 5 minutes | Cook time: 55 minutes | Serves 3-4

- 300g of sliced celery (tough strings removed)
- 2 tbsp. of olive oil
- 1 clove of garlic, peeled
- 500ml of vegetable stock
- 200g of peeled potatoes, cut in chunks
- crusty bread, for serving
- 100ml of milk

1. In a large skillet over medium heat, heat the oil, then add the celery, garlic, and potatoes and toss to coat. Cook, turning often, for 15 minutes with a splash of the water and a large teaspoon of salt, adding a little extra water if the veg starts to stick.
2. Bring the vegetable stock to a boil, then reduce to low heat and continue to cook for another 20 minutes, or till the potatoes are breaking apart & the celery is mushy. Purée the soup with a stick blender, then add the milk & blitz again. Season with salt and pepper to taste. With crusty bread, serve.

PER SERVING

Calories: 163 | Fat: 9g | Carbohydrates: 15g | Protein: 3g

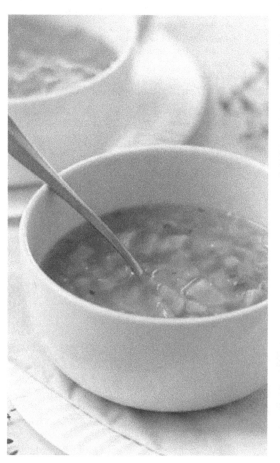

Pink Tea

Prep time: 5 minutes | Cook time: 40 minutes | Serves 2

- 2-3 ice cubes (large)
- 1 cup of water at room temperature
- 2 tbsp. of Kashmiri chai leaves
- 1 cup of water
- 2-star anise
- 2 cloves, whole (loung), optional
- 6-8 cardamom pods (green)
- 1" stick of cinnamon, optional
- 1 cup of whole milk
- 1/8 tsp. of heaped baking soda

1. Set aside ice water made from room temperature water and 2-3 huge ice cubes.
2. In a medium saucepan, heat the oil over high heat. Bring to a boil with the water, star anise, Kashmiri chai leaves, cloves, green cardamom pods, and cinnamon (if using).
3. Add baking soda after the water has reached a boil. It'll fizz up a little. Allow this solution to boil for 5-6 minutes over high heat. Use a ladle to aerate, i.e. (scoop then pour back) tea on occasion. The foam in the water will change color from light green to a rich pink. If not, add 1/8 teaspoon of baking soda. The amount of water will be drastically decreased, practically completely evaporated.
4. Pour in the ice water that has been prepared (discard any of the ice cubes). You may aerate the mixture numerous times to intensify the color if desired. Combine the milk, half-and-half, salt, and sweetener in a mixing bowl. Allow it to come to a mild boil before removing it from the heat. Allowing it to boil too long will cause it to lose part of its pink hue. Adjust the salt and sweetener to taste.
5. Strain the tea into mugs and top with crushed almonds and pistachios.

PER SERVING

Calories: 93.5 | Fat: 6.5g | Carbohydrates: 7g | Protein: 3.5g

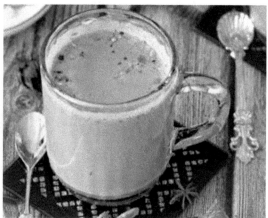

Chicken Soup

Prep time: 5 minutes | Cook time: 25 minutes | Serves 4

- ¼ cup of chopped onion
- 300 grams of chicken with bones
- 3-4 garlic cloves, whole (smashed)
- 2 bay leaves
- ¼ cup of chopped carrot
- 2-3 sprigs of thyme
- salt to taste
- 4 cups of water
- ¼ tsp. of black pepper, freshly cracked

1. 300 g bone-in chicken, well washed when making the soup, it's best to use the chicken with the bones since the bones give a lot of flavors. If bone-in chicken isn't available, use 150-200 g boneless chicken. In a pressure cooker, combine the rinsed chicken, 1/4 cup onion, 3-4 garlic cloves (smashed), 1/4 cup chopped carrot, 2-3 sprigs thyme, 2 bay leaves, and 4 cups water.
2. Season with salt and black pepper to taste, then pressure cook for 1 whistle on high heat.
3. Reduce the heat and cook for 10 to 12 minutes.
4. Turn off the heat in the pressure cooker. Allow the pressure to relax before opening the cooker lid freely.
5. Using a soup strainer, drain the soup.
6. Remove the chicken pieces, then shred them into tiny pieces, removing the bones in the process.
7. Pour the clear soup over the shredded pieces in every serving dish.
8. Serve with the spring onion greens as a garnish. Serve immediately.

PER SERVING
Calories: 172 | Fat: 11g | Carbohydrates: 2g | Protein: 14g

Pea, Cucumber & Lettuce soup

Prep time: 5 minutes | Cook time: 20 minutes | Serves 4

- A bunch of spring onions (small), roughly chopped
- 1 tsp. of rapeseed oil
- 1 roughly chopped cucumber
- 225g of frozen peas
- 1 round lettuce (large), roughly chopped
- 4 tsp. of vegetable bouillon
- 4 slices of rye bread
- 4 tbsp. of bio yogurt (optional)

1. In a kettle, bring 1.4 liters of water to a boil. In a large nonstick frying pan, heat the oil and sauté spring onions for 5 minutes, or until softened, turning regularly. Pour the boiling water over the cucumber, lettuce, and peas. Add the bouillon, cover, and cook for 10 minutes, or until the veggies are tender but brilliant green.
2. Using a hand blender, blitz the contents until it is completely smooth. Serve cold or hot with rye bread and a dollop of yogurt (if desired).

PER SERVING
Calories: 156 | Fat: 3g | Carbohydrates: 21g | Protein: 8g

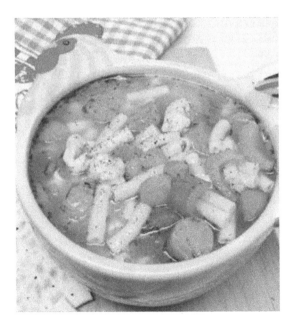

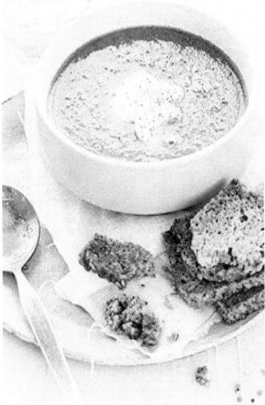

Fat-Free Broth

Prep time: 5 minutes | Cook time: 25 minutes | Serves 1

- 1 cup water for every two pounds of meat.
- The meat of choice.
- 1 Chicken Flavored Bouillon for each cup of water.

1. As usual, season your meat with salt and pepper. Put it in a big saucepan or a Crock-Pot.
2. Water should be added in proportion to the size of your meat.
3. Hand-break the chicken bouillons and pour them into the water.
4. Cover and simmer on low heat until the beef is soft and ready to eat.
5. After you've removed your meat, you'll have a lovely broth.

PER SERVING

Calories: 17 | Fat: 0g | Carbohydrates: 0.9g | Protein: 3.3g

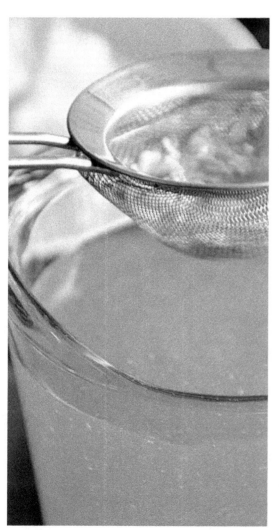

Fish and Shrimp Broth

Prep time: 5 minutes | Cook time: 30 minutes | Serves 4

- 500 grams of fish
- 250 grams of raw shrimp (with the shells)
- 2 onions
- 1 tsp. of coriander
- 1 tbsp. of vegetable oil
- 1 bay leaf
- 375 milliliters of white wine
- 125 milliliters of dry vermouth
- 1 liter of water
- 2 carrots (medium-sized)
- 2 Fennel bulb
- salt
- 1 bunch of dill
- freshly ground black pepper

1. Remove the shells from the shrimp and rinse them. Rinse the fish pieces well. Cut onions into quarters after rinsing them. In a saucepan, heat the oil. Sauté for a few minutes with the onions, shrimp shells, coriander seeds, and bay leaf. Vermouth is used to deglaze the pan. Combine the wine, water, and fish pieces in a mixing bowl. Bring to boil on low heat, then reduce to low heat and continue to cook for approximately 20 minutes.
2. Fennel should be rinsed and trimmed. Carrots should be peeled. Fennel and carrots should be finely chopped. Dill should be rinsed, shaken dry, and chopped.
3. Using a fine strainer, strain the fish broth into another pan. Salt & pepper to taste. Cook for 10 minutes after adding the veggies. Bring to a boil, then reduce to low heat and cook for 3-4 minutes, or till the shrimp are cooked through. Strain the soup & season to taste before serving, garnished with dill.

PER SERVING

Calories: 103 | Fat: 0.8g | Carbohydrates: 5g | Protein: 8.8g

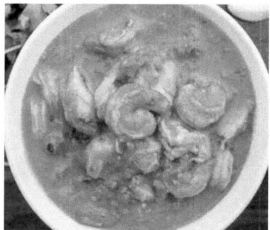

Chicken Bone healthy Broth

Prep time: 5 minutes | Cook time: 8 hours 10 minutes | Serves 12

- 2 pounds of chicken feet
- 2 and 1/2 pounds of chicken thighs on the bone
- 2 tbsp. of apple cider vinegar
- 2 roughly chopped carrots
- 1 roughly chopped onion
- 3 stalks of celery, roughly chopped
- 1 bunch of parsley rinsed well

1. In a big soup pot, combine the chicken thighs, vinegar, chicken feet, carrots, onions, and celery. Fill the pot with enough water to cover up all of the bones.
2. Allow yourself 30 mins.-1 hour of resting time. Bring to boil, then lower to low heat, cover, and cook for 6-8 hours, skimming off any scum that rises to the surface. Allow for another 10-15 minutes of simmering after adding the parsley. Allow cooling before straining the broth.
3. Keep the broth refrigerated. Remove any hardened fat from the surface.

PER SERVING

Calories: 9 | Fat: 1g | Carbohydrates: 2g | Protein: 5g

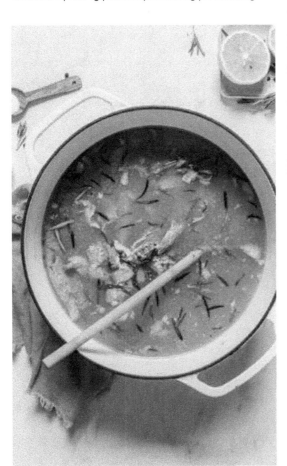

Beef Bone Mineral Rich Broth

Prep time: 5 minutes | Cook time: 12 hours 10 minutes | Serves 10

- 1 and 1/2 pounds of beef short ribs on the bone, preferably grass-fed
- 4 pounds of knucklebones and beef marrow, preferably grass-fed
- 1 and 1/2 pounds of beef neck bones, preferably grass-fed
- 3 roughly chopped onions
- 1/2 cup of apple cider vinegar (raw)
- 3 roughly chopped carrots
- 4 shitake mushrooms (dried)
- 3 stalks of celery, roughly chopped
- 10 black peppercorns
- 1 bunch of parsley washed well
- 2 bay leaves

1. Preheat the oven up to 400 degrees Fahrenheit.
2. In a large stockpot, combine the marrow and knucklebones with vinegar and enough water to cover bones. Allow for an hour of rest.
3. In a roasting pan, place neck bones and short ribs and roast for 40-45 minutes to an hour, or until beautifully browned. Add onions, celery, carrots, shitake mushrooms, peppercorns, and bay leaves to the saucepan. Fill the roasting pan halfway with water, scrape away any browned parts, and add to pot. If required, add extra water to cover all of the bones. Bring to boil, then lower to low heat and continue to cook for 12 hours at least, skimming the surface to eliminate any scum that has risen to the surface.
4. Cook for another 10-15 minutes after adding the parsley. Allow to cool before straining the broth. Save the meat and marrow from the short ribs for another time.
5. Keep the broth refrigerated. Remove any hardened fat from the surface.

PER SERVING

Calories: 27 | Fat: 1g | Carbohydrates: 6g | Protein: 1g

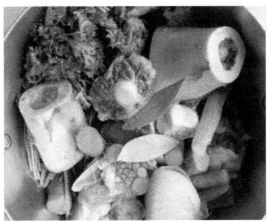

Red Lentil Lemon Soup

Prep time: 5 minutes | Cook time: 45 minutes | Serves 4

- 1 onion (large), chopped
- 3 tbsp. of olive oil, more for drizzling
- 2 cloves of garlic, minced
- 1 tsp. of ground cumin
- 1 tbsp. of tomato paste
- ¼ tsp. of kosher salt, more to taste
- Pinch of chile powder (ground) or cayenne
- ¼ tsp. of ground black pepper
- 1-quart vegetable or chicken broth
- 1 cup of red lentils
- 2 cups of water
- 1 carrot (large), diced and peeled
- 3 tbsp. of chopped fresh cilantro
- Juice of half lemon

1. 3 tablespoons oil, heated in a big saucepan over high heat till hot and shimmering Sauté the onion and garlic until golden, approximately 4 minutes.
2. Sauté for another 2 minutes after adding the cumin, tomato paste, salt, black pepper, and chili powder or cayenne.
3. Combine the broth, lentils, 2 cups of water, and carrot in a large mixing bowl. Bring to simmer, then reduce to medium-low heat with a partly covered saucepan. Simmer for 30 minutes or until lentils are tender. If required, season with salt.
4. Purée half of the soup in an immersion or a food processor or standard blender, then return it to the saucepan. The soup should have a thick texture.
5. If necessary, reheat the soup before adding the cilantro and lemon juice. Serve the soup with a drizzle of excellent olive oil and a small dusting of chili powder, if preferred.

PER SERVING

Calories: 204 | Fat: 1g | Carbohydrates: 38g | Protein: 13g

Hazelnut, Celeriac, & Truffle Soup

Prep time: 5 minutes | Cook time: 1 hour 5 minutes | Serves 6

- A small bunch of thyme
- 1 tbsp. of olive oil
- 2 bay leaves
- 1 garlic clove (fat), chopped
- 1 chopped onion
- 1 peeled celeriac (almost 1kg), chopped
- 1l vegetable stock
- 1 potato, chopped (about 200g)
- 100ml of soya cream
- 1 tbsp. of truffle oil, plus one extra drizzle for serving
- 50g of hazelnuts (blanched), toasted & roughly chopped

1. Heat the oil in a big saucepan over low heat. Using a piece of twine, tie the bay leaves and thyme sprigs together and place them in the pan with onion and a bit of salt. Cook for 10 minutes, or till softened but not browned.
2. Cook for another minute after adding the garlic, then add the potato and celeriac. Stir everything together well and then season with a generous amount of salt & white pepper. Pour in stock, bring to a boil, then reduce to a low heat and continue to cook for about 30 minutes, or until the veggies are totally soft.
3. Remove the herbs, mix in the cream, turn off the heat, and blitz until absolutely smooth. Stir in 1/2 tablespoon truffle oil at one time, tasting for seasoning — the intensity of the oil varies, so start with less and add a bit at a time.
4. To serve, reheat soup until its steaming hot, then spoon into bowls and sprinkle with hazelnuts, black pepper, and a drizzle of the truffle oil on top.

PER SERVING

Calories: 237 | Fat: 15g | Carbohydrates: 14g | Protein: 5g

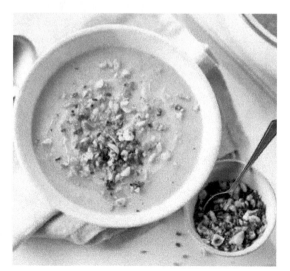

Fennel, Leek, & Potato Soup with the Cashel Blue Cheese

Prep time: 5 minutes | Cook time: 55 minutes | Serves 6

- 3 finely sliced leeks (large), trimmed and washed
- 2 heads of fennel
- 60g of butter
- 900ml of water or chicken stock
- 1 potato (large), peeled and diced
- 1 clove of garlic, sliced
- 50g of toasted walnuts
- 100ml of double cream
- 75g of crumbled Cashel Blue cheese

1. Remove the rough outer leaves & the firm core from each quarter of the fennel. Remove the remaining meat, including any of the little fronds.
2. In a saucepan, melt the butter and add the leeks, fennel, and potato. Cook for approximately 5 minutes over medium heat, flipping the veggies over in butter. Color should not be added to the veggies. Cook the veggies for 20 minutes, stirring occasionally, after adding a splash of the water and covering the pan. Season with salt and pepper, then add the water or stock and garlic. Bring to a boil, then reduce to a low heat and cover with a foyer lid.
3. Cook for 10-15 minutes, or until the vegetables are totally soft. Allow to cool after adding the cream. Blend until fully smooth in a blender. Return mixture to the pot and taste for seasoning; it may be reheated briefly just before serving. Pour into individual dishes and top with walnuts and cheese.

PER SERVING

Calories: 305 | Fat: 23g | Carbohydrates: 11g | Protein: 11g

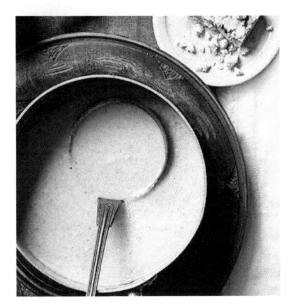

Broccoli & Leek soup with cheesy scones

Prep time: 5 minutes | Cook time: 50 minutes | Serves 4

- 400g of potatoes, peeled & cut in medium chunks
- 375g of thinly sliced leeks
- 2 chopped garlic cloves
- 340g of roughly chopped broccoli
- 2 tsp. of vegetable bouillon powder
- 250ml of milk
- 1 tsp. of baking powder
- 165g of wholemeal flour, plain
- 20g finely grated parmesan or any other vegetarian alternative
- 100ml of milk
- 1 tsp. of mustard powder
- 65g of soft goat's cheese
- ½ tbsp. of olive oil
- 4 sliced tomatoes, to serve

1. In a large pan, combine the leeks, potatoes, and garlic with the bouillon. Pour 800ml boiling water over the top, stir well, cover, and cook for 15 minutes.
2. Cover and simmer for another 5 minutes, or until the broccoli is barely tender. Blend till smooth with a hand blender, then add the milk and pulse again. If the soup seems to be excessively thick, add a little stock.
3. Preheat the oven to 220°C/200°C fan/gas 7 & line a baking pan with baking paper to prepare the scones. Combine the flour, baking powder, and all but 1 tablespoon of parmesan cheese, as well as all of the mustard powder, in a mixing bowl. Add the oil and milk in a slow, steady stream, whisking constantly using a cutlery knife till the mixture comes all together. Press the leftover parmesan on top of the log, which should be approximately 16cm long & 6cm broad. Cut each piece in half lengthwise, then in half again to make four wedge-shaped scones. Place scones on the baking sheet and bake for 10 to 12 minutes, or until golden brown.
4. Half 2 scones and top with half tomato and half the goat's cheese. Half of the soup should be ladled into 2 bowls and served with the scones. The residual soup may be kept in the refrigerator for up to 3 days.

PER SERVING

Calories: 411 | Fat: 11g | Carbohydrates: 54g | Protein: 20g

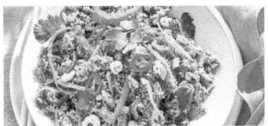

Roasted Sweet Potato, Red Pepper and Smoked Paprika Soup

Prep time: 5 minutes | Cook time: 40 minutes | Serves 2

- 1 de-seeded red pepper, cut into chunks
- 1 roughly chopped sweet potato, in dices with skin still on
- 1 peeled red onion, cut in chunks
- 1 tsp. of smoked paprika
- 3 peeled garlic cloves
- 2 tbsp. of olive oil
- 200ml of chicken stock
- 200ml of coconut milk
- 1 tsp. of maple syrup
- ½ tbsp. of Sriracha

1. Preheat the oven to 190 degrees Fahrenheit/170 degrees Fahrenheit fan/gas 5. On a baking pan, combine the pepper, sweet potato, onion, and garlic. Drizzle with oil after sprinkling with paprika and pepper. Toss everything together. Roast for 30 minutes, or until golden brown.
2. Combine the roasted vegetables, coconut milk, stock, Sriracha, and maple syrup in a blender (or you can use a stick blender). Blend until completely smooth. Return to the pan & heat until the sauce is sizzling hot. Season to taste and pour in a flask. Serve with toasted sourdough or soda bread.

PER SERVING

Calories: 491 | Fat: 33g | Carbohydrates: 36g | Protein: 9g

Ginger Lemongrass Chicken Broth

Prep time: 5 minutes | Cook time: 10 minutes | Serves 4

- 1 cut-up onion
- 1 pound of chicken thighs (organic), on bone with skin
- 1 stalk of celery cut up
- 1 tbsp. of vinegar
- 2 slices of ginger
- 2 slices of ginger
- 1 stalk of lemongrass
- Sea salt, to taste

1. In a slow cooker, combine the onion, chicken thighs, ginger, celery, and vinegar. Fill the pot with just enough water to cover the contents. Cook for 8-12 hrs. On a low heat setting, until the broth is barely boiling. Remove the soup from the pot and strain it. 4 cups rich chicken stock set aside; chill and store or freeze the remainder of the liquid for later use.
2. Lemongrass stalks and the bottom of the lemongrass bulb should be removed. Lemongrass should be crushed using a mallet. Bring 4 cups of chicken broth, lemongrass, and ginger to a boil in a saucepan. Reduce the heat to low and cook for 10 minutes. Lemongrass and ginger should be removed. Season with salt to taste.

PER SERVING

Calories: 19 | Fat: 1g | Carbohydrates: 4g | Protein: 1g

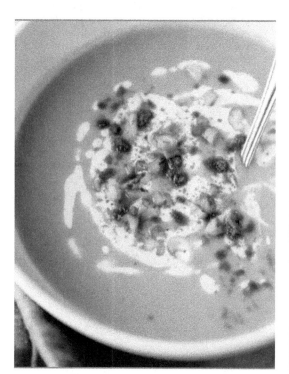

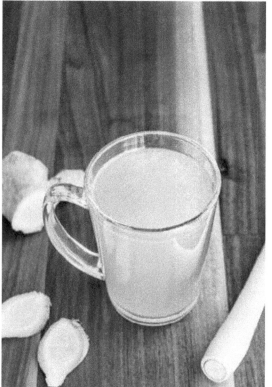

Mulligatawny soup

Prep time: 5 minutes | Cook time: 1 hour 5 minutes | Serves 4

- 20g of butter
- 2 tbsp. of olive oil
- 1 finely chopped onion
- 2 sticks of celery, chopped
- 3 peeled carrots, chopped
- 1 peeled parsnip, chopped
- 2 cloves of garlic, chopped
- 1 piece of ginger (thumb-sized), peeled and grated
- 1 cored eating apple, chopped
- 1 and ½ to 2 tbsp. of curry powder (medium)
- 1 tsp. of ground cumin
- ¼ tsp. of sweet smoked paprika
- 1.2l of hot chicken stock
- 1 tbsp. of tomato purée
- 100g of basmati rice
- 1 tbsp. of mango chutney
- ½ juiced lemon
- ½ bunch of coriander (small), shredded
- Some yogurt, to serve

1. In a casserole dish, melt the olive oil and butter and cook the celery and onion with a touch of salt for 10 to 12 minutes, or until transparent and softened. Cook for 1 minute longer after adding the carrots, garlic, parsnip, ginger, and apple. Combine the curry powder, cumin, and paprika in a mixing bowl. Season with salt and pepper after adding the tomato purée and stock. Reduce the heat to a low heat, cover, and cook for 35-40 minutes.
2. Rinse the rice then cook it in boiling water for 10 minutes. Using a blender, puree the soup until smooth. Drain rice and combine it with the lemon juice, mango chutney, and half of the coriander in the soup. Season with salt and pepper, then spoon into dishes with the rest of coriander and yogurt.

PER SERVING

Calories: 321 | Fat: 12g | Carbohydrates: 37g | Protein: 12g

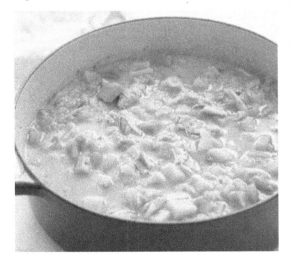

Miso Soup

Prep time: 5 minutes | Cook time: 15 minutes | Serves 4

- 1l dashi
- 5g of wakame seaweed (dried)
- 200g of silken tofu (fresh), or firm, cut in 1cm cubes
- 3 tbsp. of red miso paste
- 2 tbsp. of white miso paste
- finely chopped spring onions, to serve

1. Place the wakame into a small bowl with cold water and let aside for 5 minutes, or until the leaves are fully expanded.
2. Make the dashi or heat till it reaches the rolling boil (see tip below). Cook for 1 minute before adding the tofu and seaweed.
3. Turn down the heat. Dip a strainer or ladle into the saucepan with both kinds of miso. Inside the strainer or ladle, carefully loosen the miso paste with a spoon; the paste will gradually melt in the dashi. Turn off the heat as soon as all of the miso has dissolved into the broth. To add color and scent, scatter chopped spring onions over top.

PER SERVING

Calories: 99 | Fat: 4g | Carbohydrates: 9g | Protein: 7g

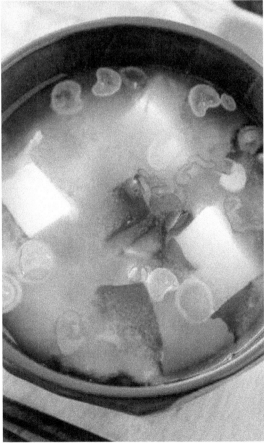

Sage & Butternut Squash Soup
Prep time: 5 minutes | Cook time: 1 hour | Serves 8

- 1 tbsp. of butter
- 1 tbsp. of olive oil
- 3 chopped onions
- 1.4kg of peeled, butternut squash, deseeded
- 2 tbsp. of chopped sage
- 1 tbsp. of clear honey
- A bunch of chives, snipped
- Black pepper, to serve
- 1 and ½ l of vegetable stock

1. In a large pot or flameproof casserole, melt the butter and oil. Cook, stirring occasionally, until the sage and onions are completely soft, approximately 15 minutes. Add the squash and simmer for 5 minutes, stirring occasionally. Bring the stock and honey to a low boil, then reduce to a low heat and cook till the squash is soft.
2. Allow the soup to cool slightly so you don't burn yourself, then puree with a hand blender or in stages in a blender until completely smooth. Season with salt and pepper, then thin with a little more water or stock if soup is too thick. Sprinkle with cracked black pepper and chives before serving.

PER SERVING
Calories: 130 | Fat: 4g | Carbohydrates: 21g | Protein: 3g

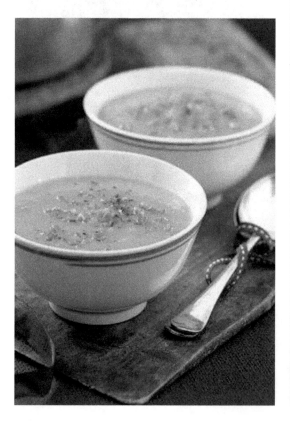

Potato & Minty Pea Soup
Prep time: 5 minutes | Cook time: 30 minutes | Serves 4

- 1 chopped onion
- 2 tsp. of vegetable oil
- 800g of peeled potato, cut in small chunks
- 350g of frozen pea
- 1l of vegetable stock
- handful of mint, chopped

1. In a big saucepan, heat the oil and cook the onion for 4-5 minutes, or until softened. Bring the stock and potatoes to a boil, then remove from the heat. Cover and cook for 10-15 minutes, or until the peas are cooked, adding them 2 minutes before the end of cooking time.
2. Remove a fourth of the veggies from the pan using a slotted spoon and put aside. With a hand blender or in a food processor, puree the remaining veggies and stock until smooth, then toss in the saved vegetables, chopped mint, and spices. Serve with a side of toast.

PER SERVING
Calories: 249 | Fat: 3g | Carbohydrates: 48g | Protein: 11g

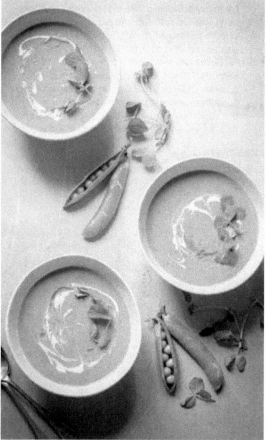

Cauliflower & Spiced parsnip soup

Prep time: 5 minutes | Cook time: 1 hour 5 minutes | Serves 6-8

- 1 cauliflower (medium), cut into florets
- 1 tbsp. of olive oil
- 3 chopped parsnips
- 1 tbsp. of fennel seed
- 2 chopped onions
- 1 tsp. of coriander seed
- 3 sliced garlic cloves
- ½ tsp. of turmeric
- 1-2 deseeded green chilies, chopped
- juice and zest of 1 lemon
- 5cm piece of ginger, sliced
- handful of coriander, chopped
- 1 l of vegetable stock

1. In a large saucepan, heat the oil and add the veggies. Cover partly with plastic wrap and let to sweat for 10-15 minutes, or until tender but not brown. Dry-roast the spices in a separate pan with a bit of salt for some minutes until aromatic. To make a fine powder, use a pestle and mortar.
2. Cook for approximately 5 minutes, stirring often, after adding the garlic, chili, ginger, and spices to the veggies. Combine the juice and lemon zest in a mixing bowl. Pour in stock and fill up as needed to barely cover the vegetables. Cook for another 25-30 minutes, or until all of the veggies are soft.
3. Blend until completely smooth. If necessary, add additional water to thin the consistency until you have a thick but pourable soup. Season liberally with salt and pepper, then toss in coriander and additional lemon juice to taste. Eat right quickly or keep refrigerated to reheat. This freezes wonderfully as well. If desired, serve with crusty bread.

PER SERVING

Calories: 133 | Fat: 4g | Carbohydrates: 18g | Protein: 7g

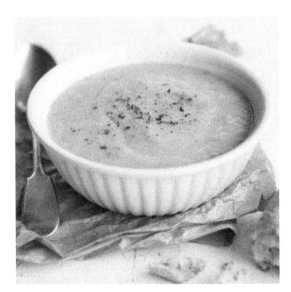

Spiced Moroccan cauliflower and almond soup

Prep time: 5 minutes | Cook time: 30 minutes | Serves 4

- 2 tbsp. of olive oil
- 1 cauliflower (large)
- ½ tsp. of each ground cinnamon, coriander and cumin
- 1 l of hot chicken or vegetable stock
- 2 tbsp. of harissa paste, plus some extra drizzle
- 50g of flaked almond (toasted), plus some extra to serve

1. Cauliflower should be cut into tiny florets. In a large pan, heat the ground cinnamon, olive oil, cumin, and coriander, as well as the harissa paste, for 2 minutes. Combine the cauliflower, stock, and almonds in a large mixing bowl.
2. Cook, covered, for 20 minutes, or until cauliflower is soft. Blend until smooth, then top with a sprinkling of toasted almonds and a drizzle of harissa.

PER SERVING

Calories: 200 | Fat: 16g | Carbohydrates: 8g | Protein: 8g

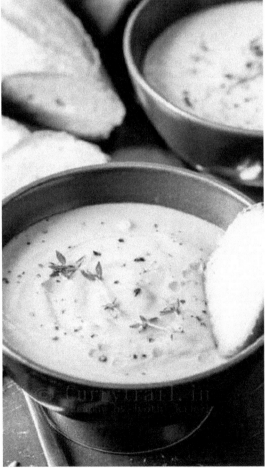

Gruyere, Broccoli & chorizo soup

Prep time: 5 minutes | Cook time: 42 minutes | Serves 6

- 1 tbsp. of fennel seeds
- 1 tbsp. of yellow mustard seeds
- 150g of chorizo (skin removed), cut in cubes
- 1 chopped onion
- 1 tbsp. of rapeseed oil
- 2 cloves of garlic, chopped
- 2 broccoli heads (approx. 800g), cut in florets
- 1 and ½ l of chicken stock
- 3 tbsp. of double cream
- 150g of gruyere, grated

1. Over medium heat, dry-fry the fennel and mustard seeds till the mustard seeds begin to burst. Grind seeds to a powder form in a pestle and mortar.
2. Fry chorizo (without any oil) in a big pot for 4 minutes over medium heat till it released its oils, then move it to a dish using a slotted spoon and put aside.
3. Add the garlic and onion to the pan with the oil. Cook, stirring occasionally, for 10 minutes, or till the onion is soft. Before adding the chicken stock and broccoli, toss in ground spice mix & cook for another minute, stirring constantly. Bring liquid to a boil, then cover the pan, reduce the heat to low, and cook for 5 minutes, or till the broccoli is soft.
4. In the food processor or using a stick blender, puree the soup until totally smooth, then whisk in 2-3rds of the gruyere as well as the cream. Season with salt and pepper to taste. Fill dishes halfway with the soup and top it with the leftover cheese and chorizo.

PER SERVING

Calories: 392 | Fat: 28g | Carbohydrates: 7g | Protein: 26g

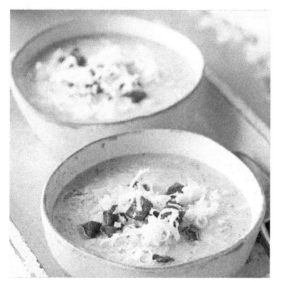

Tomato & Carrot soup

Prep time: 5 minutes | Cook time: 1 hour 30 minutes | Serves 8

- 2 chopped onions
- 3 tbsp. of olive oil
- 2 chopped celery sticks
- 250g of floury potato, diced
- 1 and ¼ kg of carrot, sliced
- 5 bay leaves (dried or fresh)
- 750g of cherry tomato
- 500g of carton passata
- 2 cubes of vegetable stock
- 1 tbsp. of red wine vinegar
- 1 tbsp. of sugar (granulated or caster)
- 250ml of whole milk

1. In your biggest saucepan, slowly simmer the oil, onions, and celery until softened. Add the potatoes and carrots and cook for a few minutes, then add the rest of the ingredients, except the milk, along with 1 liter of water. Bring to a low boil, then reduce to a low heat. Cover and cook for 30 minutes, then uncover and cook for another 20-30 minutes.
2. Remove bay leaves and puree the soup using a hand blender until smooth. Pour in the milk and same amount of water as necessary. Season with salt and pepper to taste, then reheat through. Make ahead and refrigerate for up to 2 days, or freeze for up to 1 month and reheat gently.

PER SERVING

Calories: 175 | Fat: 7g | Carbohydrates: 24g | Protein: 5g

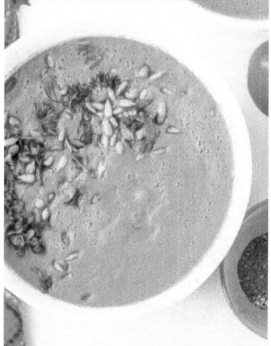

Spinach Soup
Prep time: 5 minutes | Cook time: 35 minutes | Serves 4

- 1 bunch of spring onions, chopped
- 25g of butter
- 1 leek, sliced (about 120g)
- 1 potato, small (about 200g), peeled & diced
- 2 sticks of celery, sliced (about 85g)
- ½ tsp. of ground black pepper
- 2 bags of spinach (200-235g)
- 1 l stock (prepared with 2 vegetable or chicken stock cubes)
- 150g of crème fraiche (half-fat)

1. In a large pot, melt the butter. Combine the leek, spring onions, celery, and potato in a large mixing bowl. Stir well and cover with a lid. Cook for 10 min, stirring occasionally.
2. Pour in the liquid and heat until potato is mushy, about 10 to 15 minutes.
3. Cook for a few minutes, until the spinach has wilted. Blitz the soup with a hand blender until it is smooth.
4. Pour in crème fraiche and mix well. Serve after reheating.

PER SERVING
Calories: 192 | Fat: 12.6g | Carbohydrates: 13.1g | Protein: 6.5g

Cardamom & Lentil soup
Prep time: 5 minutes | Cook time: 25 minutes | Serves 2-3

- 2 garlic cloves (fat), crushed
- 1 onion (large), finely chopped
- 1 carrot (large), finely chopped
- 2 tbsp. of oil, rapeseed, sunflower, or groundnut
- A piece of ginger (thumb-sized), peeled & finely chopped
- ½ tsp. of turmeric
- 1 tsp. of cumin, ground or seeds
- seeds from ten cardamom pods
- 100g of red lentils
- juice and zest of 1 lemon
- 400ml can of light coconut milk
- handful of coriander or parsley, chopped
- A pinch of chili flakes

1. To soften the garlic, onion, carrot, & ginger, place them in a pot with the oil & heat for some minutes. Combine the cardamom, turmeric, and cumin in a bowl. Cook, stirring constantly, for some minutes longer, until spices are fragrant.
2. In the same pan, add lentils. Pour coconut milk on top, then pour the water from the can. Bring to a boil, then lower to a low heat and cook for 15 minutes, or until lentils are swelled and soft but still have a bite to them. Pulse your soup with a hand blender until part of it is totally pureed, leaving some bigger vegetable bits.
3. Zest lemon directly into pan, then pour the juice on the soup & season to taste with salt, pepper, and herbs. Pour into the bowls and top with a bit extra lemon zest.

PER SERVING
Calories: 363 | Fat: 20g | Carbohydrates: 31g | Protein: 11g

Curried parsnip, lentil, & apple soup
Prep time: 5 minutes | Cook time: 1 hour | Serves 6-8

- 3 tbsp. of medium curry paste
- 2 tbsp. of sunflower oil
- 2 onions (medium), roughly chopped
- 140g of dried red lentils
- 500g of parsnips (around five medium parsnips), peeled & cut in chunks
- 2 (about 400g) Bramley apples, peeled and cored, cut in chunks
- natural yogurt, for serving (optional)
- 1 and ½ l chicken or vegetable stock, made with one stock cube
- coriander (chopped), to serve (optional)

1. In a big saucepan, heat the oil. Stir the onions and curry paste together for 3 minutes over medium heat. Combine the parsnips, lentils, and apple chunks in a large mixing bowl. Bring the stock to a simmer after pouring it in. Reduce the heat to low and simmer, stirring periodically, for 30 minutes, or until parsnips are too soft as well as the lentils are mushy.
2. Remove from heat and mix until smooth using a stick blender. (Alternatively, let it cool for some minutes before blending in the food processor.) Season with salt and pepper to taste.
3. Gently heat through, then ladle into large dishes. Serve with a dollop of natural yogurt and a sprinkling of fresh coriander, if desired.

PER SERVING
Calories: 204 | Fat: 5g | Carbohydrates: 24g | Protein: 12g

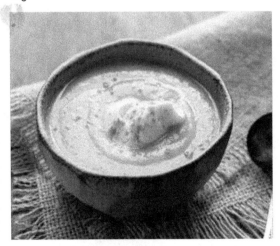

Chapter 9
Snacks

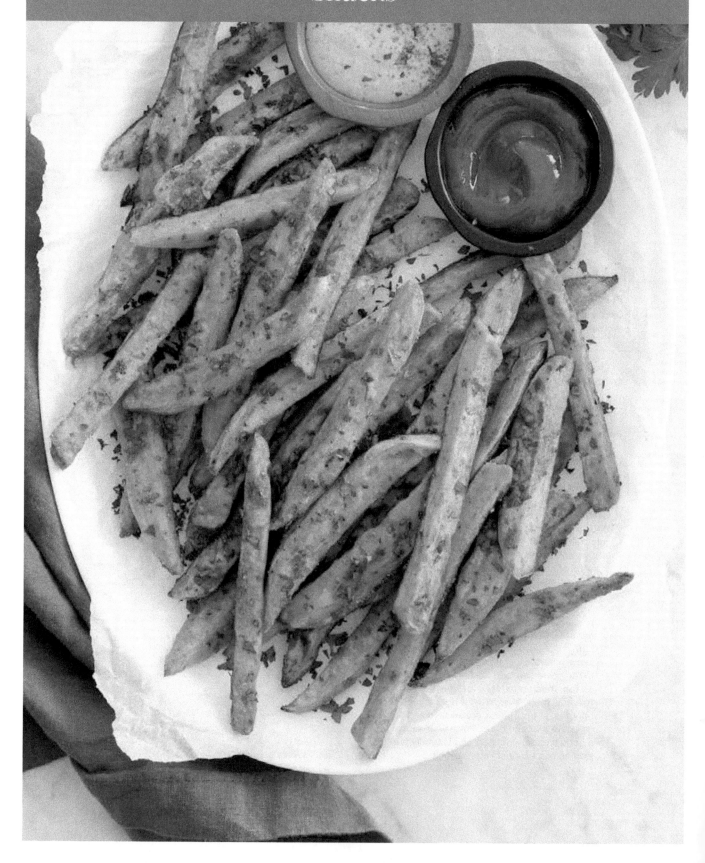

Sweet Potato Fries

Prep time: 5 minutes | Cook time: 40 minutes | Serves 4

- 2 tbsp. of cornstarch or potato starch
- 1 pound of sweet potatoes
- 3 tbsp. of vegetable oil
- 1/2 tsp. of kosher salt

1. Preheat the oven up to 400 degrees Fahrenheit. Preheat the oven to 400°F and split it into thirds using two racks. If preferred, line two rimmed baking sheets with the parchment paper.
2. The sweet potato should be peeled and chopped into small pieces. Cut longitudinally in half. Cut longitudinally into 1/4-inch wide boards after turning onto the cut side. Cut the boards lengthwise into 1/4-inch thick sticks or wedges by laying them flat.
3. Using a pastry brush, coat sweet potato into starch. Put the sweet potato in a big dish or zip-top plastic bag, add the cornstarch or potato starch and salt, and toss or shake until the starch is completely absorbed.
4. Using a brush, coat sweet potato in oil. Toss in the oil, then toss well to coat.
5. Place 2 baking sheets on top of each other. Spread the sweet potato across the two baking sheets in a single, equal layer, allowing room around each fry.
6. Roast. Roast for 15 minutes, or until some fries are just beginning to brown all around the edges. Preheat the oven to 350°F. Take the baking sheets out from the oven. Flip sweet potatoes with a turner or flat spatula. Return to the oven, swapping the sheets in between racks, and roast for another 5 to 15 minutes, or till the fries are soft on the inside & crispy on the exterior. As they cool, they would crisp up a bit more.
7. Season to taste and serve. Before serving, season with some more salt if required.

PER SERVING

Calories: 206 | Fats: 10.6g | Carbohydrates: 26.5g | Proteins: 1.8g.

Ale Pie and Steak with Mushrooms

Prep time: 5 minutes | Cook time: 1 hour 25 minutes | Serves 8

- 1 diced onion
- 1 and ¼ pounds of beef stew meat, cubed
- 1 can of pale ale or lager beer (12 fluid ounces)
- ½ tsp. of dried thyme
- 2 cloves of garlic, minced
- 1 and ½ tsp. of fresh parsley, chopped
- Some salt and black pepper to taste
- 2 tbsp. of Worcestershire sauce
- 2 cups of peeled potatoes, cubed
- 1 tbsp. of all-purpose flour
- 1 pastry for pie, double-crust
- 1 and ½ cups of fresh mushrooms, quartered

1. In a large saucepan, combine the onion, beef stew meat, and ale. Simmer for 30 minutes over low heat or till the meat is tender.
2. Garlic, parsley, thyme, salt, Worcestershire sauce, and black pepper are used to season the meat. Combine the mushrooms and potatoes in a mixing bowl. Cover and cook over medium heat for 10 to 15 minutes, or till potatoes are just soft enough to cut with a fork. In a small mixing bowl, combine a tiny quantity of the sauce with the flour, and mix into the meat. Simmer until the sauce has thickened somewhat.
3. In a 9-inch pie pan, press one pie crust in the bottom and up to the sides. Fill the crust with the mixture of hot beef and top with the remaining pie crust. To vent steam, cut slits in the top crust and crimp the sides to bind them together.
4. Bake for 35 to 40 minutes in a preheated oven till the crust is brownish golden and the gravy is bubbling.

PER SERVING

Calories: 473 | Fats: 28.7g | Carbohydrates: 32.4g | Proteins: 17.5g.

Baked Sweet Potato

Prep time: 5 minutes | Cook time: 30-45 minutes | Serves 4

- Some Vegetable oil
- 4 Sweet potatoes

1. Preheat the oven to 350°F and wash sweet potatoes as follows: Preheat the oven to 375 degrees Fahrenheit. Scrub sweet potatoes well and dry them with a paper towel.
2. Lubricate them: Prepare aluminum foil squares for as many of the sweet potatoes as you want to roast. Drizzle a tiny quantity of vegetable oil over each potato on a foil square. Apply a thin, uniform coating of oil to the potatoes using your hands.
3. Prick with a fork, cover in plastic wrap, and roast: Using a fork, prick each of the sweet potatoes many times and cover loosely in foil. Make sure that the foil is very well-sealed before using it. Place them on a baking pan and roast them in the oven.
4. Check for the doneness: Based on the size of the potatoes, they may take anywhere from 30 minutes to an hour to cook. Squeeze one of the potatoes in the oven mitt-protected hand and put a fork or sharp knife into the middle after 30 minutes. They should be rather soft, and the knife must slide smoothly through them. If not, return it to the oven for another 10 minutes and check again.
5. Whether you want to savor it right now or keep it for later, the choice is you may eat your sweet potatoes right now or keep them in the fridge for later. They'll last a few days in the fridge. Reheat in the toaster oven or microwave as required, or use in recipes.

PER SERVING

Calories: 160 | Fats: 0.8 g | Carbohydrates: 32.5 g | Proteins: 5.8 g

Roasted Honey Parsnips

Prep time: 5 minutes | Cook time: 55 minutes | Serves 8

- 1 tbsp. of flour
- 500g of parsnips
- 1 tbsp. of honey
- 2 tbsp. of butter
- 2 tbsp. of sunflower oil

1. Take 500g parsnips, top and tail, and cut any bigger ones in half lengthwise, then place in a large pot with salted water, then bring to a boil, and simmer for 5 minutes.
2. Preheat oven to 190°C/170°C fan forced/gas 5
3. Toss the parsnips with 1 tablespoon flour and 1 tablespoon honey.
4. Combine the parsnips, 2 tbsp. of sunflower oil, 2 tbsp. of butter and spices in a roasting pan.
5. Cook for 40 minutes, rotating halfway through, until golden brown.

PER SERVING

Calories: 119 | Fats: 7 g | Carbohydrates: 11 g | Proteins: 1 g

Crispy Roasted Potatoes

Prep time: 5 minutes | Cook time: 35 minutes | Serves 6-8

- 1 and ½ kg of potatoes, peelings reserved and cut in quarters
- 4 tbsp. of rapeseed oil
- 50g of butter
- 6 cloves of garlic, lightly bashed
- ½ lemon thyme bunch
- 1 tbsp. of sea salt

1. Preheat oven to 220°C/200°C fan/gas 8. To heat up the oil, pour it onto a big flameproof baking pan and place it in the oven.
2. Bring a big saucepan of the salted water to a boil, then add the potatoes and peelings (for added flavor) and continue to cook for 8-10 minutes. Remove the peelings from the potatoes and drain them. Allow for a 15-minute steaming period before returning the potatoes to the pan, covering them with the lid, and gently shaking to roughen the edges.
3. Remove tray from oven and place it over medium heat on your stove-top. Add butter to the heated oil and, with tongs, delicately flip the potatoes in the fat while allowing a little space in between them.
4. Preheat the oven up to 200 degrees Fahrenheit/180 degrees Fahrenheit fan/gas 6. Sprinkle the garlic and lemon thyme over the potatoes. Return to the oven and roast for 1 hour, turning once or twice, until golden and crisp, till sea salt has been sprinkled on top.

PER SERVING

Calories: 233 | Fats: 11g | Carbohydrates: 29g | Proteins: 3g

Sweet Potatoes Soup with Ginger and Miso

Prep time: 5 minutes | Cook time: 30 minutes | Serves 4-6

FOR SOUP:

- 1 yellow onion (large), chopped
- Olive oil
- 4 cloves of garlic, minced
- 3 cups of mashed sweet potato (from almost 3 roasted sweet potatoes)
- 1 piece of peeled fresh ginger (2-inch, about 1/4 cup), thinly sliced
- 3 tbsp. of light miso
- 1/2 cup of whole milk
- 4 cups of vegetable or chicken broth
- Salt and black pepper
- For spiced yogurt drizzle:
- 1/2 tsp. of garam masala
- 1/2 cup of whole milk yogurt
- 1/2 tbsp. of maple syrup

1. Over medium heat, cook the garlic and onion in olive oil until tender and translucent. Increase the heat slightly and stir in the ginger. Cook until the ginger is aromatic but without browning the onions and garlic. Cook till the puree is warmed, then add the miso and sweet potato mash.
2. Stir in the broth until it is evenly distributed across the pan. Bring the soup to a simmer and cover, reduce the heat, and cook for approximately 5 minutes to blend the flavors. Remove from the heat and purée with the immersion blender or in a blender.
3. Return to low heat and whisk in the milk. Season with salt and black pepper to taste. If soup is very thick, add a bit more milk until it reaches the desired consistency.
4. Combine the garam masala, yogurt, and maple syrup in a mixing bowl. To serve, drizzle the dressing over sweet potato soup.

PER SERVING

Calories: 158 | Fats: 6.1g | Carbohydrates: 23.0g | Proteins: 4.0g.

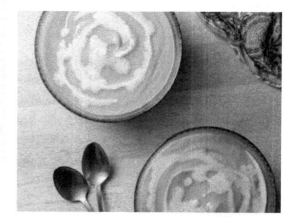

Lime-Cilantro Sardine Salad into Avocado Halves
Prep time: 5 minutes | Cook time: 20 minutes |Serves 2

- 2 tbsp. of finely chopped cilantro
- 1 can of skinless, boneless sardines packed in the oil (3.75-ounce), drained
- 1 tbsp. of mayonnaise
- 1 avocado, ripe
- 1 tbsp. of lime juice (fresh), divided
- Salad greens, to serve (optional)
- Salt and black pepper

1. Combine the cilantro, sardines, mayonnaise, and 2 and 1/2 tablespoons lime juice in a small bowl. With a fork, thoroughly combine the ingredients and season them to taste with black pepper and a sprinkle of salt, if desired.
2. Remove the pit from the avocado and cut it in half lengthwise. Scoop each of the avocado halves from its shell using a big spoon with a shallow, wide bowl: slide the tip of the spoon along the edge of avocado to loosen it, and then dip the spoon between the peel and flesh.
3. Working from the broader to the smaller end of the avocado, keep the back of a spoon as near to the skin as possible. The leftover 1/2 tsp. Lime juice should be rubbed into each half.
4. To serve, spoon half of the sardine salad into each avocado's hollow. If preferred, serve on dressed salad greens.

PER SERVING
Calories: 163 | Fats: 13.2g | Carbohydrates: 4.8g | Proteins: 7.6g

Ricotta & Cannellini Salad
Prep time: 15 minutes | Cook time: 5 minutes |Serves 6

- 2 tablespoons plain yogurt (low-fat)
- 3 tablespoons extra virgin olive oil
- 2 tablespoons fresh lemon juice
- 3/4 teaspoon oregano (ground)
- 1 tablespoon fresh mint (shredded)
- 2 (14-ounce) cans of white cannellini beans (drained and rinsed)
- 1/2 cup red onions (thinly sliced)
- 3 medium tomatoes (seeded and chopped)
- 1/4 cup Greek olives (pitted)
- 1/2 cup ricotta cheese (crumbled)
- 2 cups spinach leaves

1. In a large bowl, combine yogurt, olive oil, lemon juice, oregano, and mint; whisk well.
2. Refrigerate for at least one hour. Serve on a bed of spinach.

PER SERVING
Calories: 160 | Fat: 11g | Carbohydrates: 10g | Fiber: 2g | Protein: 6g

3 Ingredient Sugar-Free Gelatin
Prep time: 5 minutes | Cook time: 4 hours |Serves 6-8

- ¼ cup water (room temperature)
- 1 tablespoon gelatin
- 1 cup orange juice (unsweetened)

1. Combine your gelatin and room temperature water, stirring until fully dissolved.
2. Stir in your hot water, then leave to rest for about 2 minutes.
3. Add in your juice and stir until combined.
4. Transfer to serving size containers, then place on a tray in the refrigerator to set for about 4 hours.
5. Enjoy!

PER SERVING
Calories: 17 | Fat: 0g | Carbohydrates: 4g | Fiber: 0g | Protein: 0g

Cranberry Kombucha Jell-O
Prep time: 5 minutes | Cook time: 4 hours |Serves 6

- ¼ cup water (room temperature)
- ¼ cup hot water
- 1 cup cranberry kombucha (unsweetened)

1. Combine your gelatin and room temperature water, stirring until fully dissolved.
2. Stir in your hot water, then leave to rest for about 2 minutes.
3. Add in your kombucha and stir until combined.
4. Transfer to serving size containers, then place on a tray in the refrigerator to set for about 4 hours.
5. Enjoy!

PER SERVING
Calories: 13 | Fat: 0g | Carbohydrates: 1g | Fiber: 0g | Protein: 0g

Strawberry Gummies
Prep time: 5 minutes | Cook time: 4 hours |Serves 20-40

- 1 cup strawberries (hulled, chopped)
- 2 tablespoons gelatin

1. Set your water and berries on to boil on high heat. Remove from heat as soon as the mixture begins to boil.
2. Transfer to your blender and blend. Add in your gelatin, then blend once more.
3. Pour your mixture into a silicone gummy mold.
4. Place on a tray in the refrigerator to set for about 4 hours.
5. Enjoy!

PER SERVING
Calories: 3 | Fat: 0g | Carbohydrates: 0g | Fiber: 0g | Protein: 0g3

Fruity Jell-O Stars
Prep time: 15 minutes | Cook time: 5 minutes | Serves 4

- 1 tablespoon gelatin (powdered)
- ¾ cup boiling water
- 3 ½ fruit
- 1 tablespoon honey
- 1 teaspoon lemon juice

1. Add all your ingredients into your blender and blend. Add in your gelatin, then blend once more.
2. Pour your mixture into a silicone gummy mold.
3. Place on a tray in the refrigerator to set for about 4 hours.
4. Enjoy!

PER SERVING

Calories: 73 | Fat: 2g | Carbohydrates: 14g | Fiber: 0g | Protein: 1g

Plum and Nectarine Gelatin Pudding
Prep time: 15 minutes | Cook time: 5 minutes | Serves 5

- 1 nectarine (large)
- 2 plums (small)
- 2 tablespoons gelatin
- 1 ½ cup water (room temp.)
- 2 cups boiling water
- 2 teaspoons lemon juice
- 1/3 cup honey
- 1 tablespoon vanilla
- 1/8 teaspoon sea salt

1. Add your fruits in your blend to puree until smooth with room temperature water, lemon juice, and vanilla until smooth.
2. Strain through a fine-mesh strainer.
3. Combine your gelatin and fruit mixture, stirring until fully dissolved.
4. Stir in your hot water, then leave to rest for about 2 minutes.
5. Add in your remaining ingredients and stir until combined.
6. Transfer to serving size containers, then place on a tray in the refrigerator to set for about 4 hours. Enjoy!

PER SERVING

Calories: 157 | Fat: 5g | Carbohydrates: 26g | Fiber: 1g | Protein: 3g

Homemade Lemon Gelatin
Prep time: 2 hours 5 minutes | Cook time: 5 minutes | Serves 8

- 3 tablespoons gelatin (granulated)
- 1½ cup stevia
- 1 1/2 cup boiling water
- 3 cups Room temperature Water
- 1 1/8 cup Lemon Juice
- ½ teaspoon Lemon zest

1. Combine your gelatin and room temperature water, stirring until fully dissolved.
2. Stir in your hot water, then leave to rest for about 2 minutes.
3. Add in your remaining ingredients and stir until combined.
4. Transfer to serving size containers, then place on a tray in the refrigerator to set for about 4 hours. Enjoy!

PER SERVING

Calories: 68 | Fat: 0g | Carbohydrates: 1g | Fiber: 0g | Protein: 2g

Sour Blueberry Gummies
Prep time: 5 minutes | Cook time: 5 minutes | Serves 9

- 1 ½ cup blueberries
- 1/3 cup gelatin (grass-fed)
- Water

1. Set your water and berries on to boil on high heat. Remove from heat as soon as the mixture begins to boil.
2. Transfer to your blender and blend. Add in your gelatin, then blend once more.
3. Pour your mixture into a silicone gummy mold.
4. Place on a tray in the refrigerator to set for about 4 hours. Enjoy!

PER SERVING

Calories: 73 | Fat: 2g | Carbohydrates: 14g | Fiber: 0g | Protein: 1g

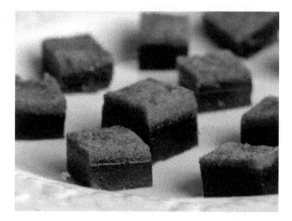

Sugar-Free Cinnamon Jelly

Prep time: 2 hours 15 minutes | Cook time: 5 minutes | Serves 2

- 1 cup room temperature water
- 2 teaspoons gelatin
- 1/2 cup apple Juice

1. Combine your gelatin and room temperature water, stirring until fully dissolved.
2. Stir in your hot water, then leave to rest for about 2 minutes.
3. Add in your apple juice and stir until combined.
4. Transfer to serving size containers, then place on a tray in the refrigerator to set for about 4 hours.
5. Enjoy!

PER SERVING

Calories: 35 | Fat: 0g | Carbohydrates: 17g | Fiber: 0g | Protein: 0g

Bean and Tomato Salad

Prep time: 10 minutes | Cook time: 5 minutes | Serves 4

- 4 medium tomatoes (seeded and chopped)
- 2 (14-ounce) cans garbanzos (drained and rinsed)
- 1/4 cup red onions (chopped finely)
- 1 cup Italian parsley (chopped finely)
- 2 tablespoons lemon juice
- 1/4 cup extra virgin olive oil
- 1/2 teaspoon salt

1. Combine your parsley, onions, beans, and tomato. Set aside. In another bowl, whisk together salt, olive oil, and lemon juice.
2. Pour dressing over vegetables. Mix and serve.

PER SERVING

Calories: 201 | Fat: 14g | Carbohydrates: 18g | Fiber: 4g | Protein: 4g

String Bean Potato Salad

Prep time: 15 minutes | Cook time: 7 minutes | Serves 4-6

- 1 1/2 lbs. string beans (slender)
- 6 small red potatoes (unpeeled, cubed)
- 1 small red onion (thinly sliced lengthwise)
- 1/3 cup extra virgin olive oil
- 1/4 cup red wine vinegar
- 1/4 cup rice vinegar
- 1 tablespoon garlic salt
- 1 teaspoon sugar

1. In a pot of boiling water, cook potatoes and string beans for about 7 minutes.
2. Drain the contents and run cold water on the beans only to stop the cooking process. Drain and set it aside.
3. In a large salad bowl, combine beans, potatoes, and onions. For the dressing, in a bowl, whisk together olive oil, vinegar, garlic salt, and sugar.
4. Toss the vegetables and dressing together until coated. Refrigerate one hour prior to serving.

PER SERVING

Calories: 142 | Fat: 11g | Carbohydrates: 10g | Fiber: 1g | Protein: 1g

Cucumber Peach Salad

Prep time: 30 minutes | Cook time: 5 minutes | Serves 4

- 2 large avocados (pitted and diced)
- 1 peach (unpeeled, pitted, and diced)
- 1 gala pear (unpeeled, cored, and diced)
- 1 cup cantaloupe (chopped)
- 1 shallot (chopped finely)
- 1 English cucumber (chopped)
- 1/4 cup fresh lime juice
- 1/4 cup fresh mint (chopped)
- 8 large lettuce leaves

1. In a medium bowl, combine all ingredients except the lettuce leaves. Sprinkle the mint and lime juice.
2. Toss until combined. Let the salad sit for at least 10–20 minutes. Serve over 2 leaves of lettuce per serving.

PER SERVING

Calories: 182 | Fat: 11g | Carbohydrates: 23g | Fiber: 3g | Protein: 6g

Strawberry & Apple Salad

Prep time: 10 minutes | Cook time: 5 minutes | Serves 2

- 1½ cup ripe strawberries
- 1½ cup Fresh apple (cut in small cubes)
- 12 Brazil nuts (blanched and thinly sliced)
- 4 tablespoonfuls lemon juice
- 7 large lettuce leaves
- 1 tablespoonful dressing

1. Cut the apples and strawberries and add Brazil nuts that have been marinated in lemon juice.
2. Shape your lettuce into a rose, and fill the lettuce with the mixture above, and cover with a spoonful salad dressing.

PER SERVING

Calories: 184 | Fat: 11g | Carbohydrates: 23g | Fiber: 4g | Protein: 4g

Bean and Couscous Salad

Prep time: 15 minutes | Cook time: 5 minutes | Serves 4

- 1 cup couscous
- 1 1/2 cup boiling water
- 1 cup sweet yellow peppers (seeded and chopped)
- 2 cups black beans (cooked)
- 1 small onion (chopped)
- 2 cups tomatoes (seeded and chopped)
- 2 medium garlic cloves (minced)
- 1/2 cup rice vinegar
- 1/4 cup olive oil
- 1/2 teaspoon salt

1. In a large bowl, place the couscous with boiling water. Cover and wait until the couscous has absorbed all the water.
2. Place couscous in a bowl and add the remaining ingredients. Mix well. Serve.

PER SERVING

Calories: 637 | Fat: 15g | Carbohydrates: 101g | Fiber: 18g | Protein: 28g

Asian Chicken Salad

Prep time: 15 minutes | Cook time: 5 minutes | Serves 1

- 1 cup romaine lettuce (chopped)
- 1 carrot (shredded)
- 1 celery (sliced thinly)
- 1/4 cup red pepper (seeded, sliced thinly)
- 1/2 cup chicken breast (cooked, cut into strips)
- 1/4 cup mangos (chopped)
- 2 tablespoons lime and ginger dressing

1. Toss together all ingredients in a medium bowl until combined.
2. Serve alone or with whole wheat bread slices.

PER SERVING

Calories: 384 | Fat: 4g | Carbohydrates: 68g | Fiber: 10g | Protein: 25g

Almond Salad

Prep time: 10 minutes | Cook time: 5 minutes | Serves 1

- 1½ cup blanched almonds (chopped)
- 18 olives
- 1½ cup celery (cut fine)
- 1 tablespoon salad dressing
- 5 medium lettuce leaves

1. Stone and chop the olives.
2. Add the almonds and the celery.
3. Mix with salad dressing and serve on the lettuce.

PER SERVING

Calories: 101 | Fat: 6g | Carbohydrates: 10g | Fiber: 3g | Protein: 2g

Vegetarian Nuttolene Salad

Prep time: 10 minutes | Cook time: 5 minutes | Serves 1

- ¼ lb. nuttolene (chopped)
- 2/3 cup celery (chopped)
- ½ lb. protose (chopped)
- 1 small teaspoonful onion (grated)
- 2 lemons juice
- Salt
- 2 tablespoonfuls mayonnaise

1. Mix all the ingredients together, then add the mayonnaise dressing last.
2. Serve

PER SERVING

Calories: 55 | Fat: 0g | Carbohydrates: 12g | Fiber: 3g | Protein: 2g

Nutty Green Salad

Prep time: 5 minutes | Cook time: 5 minutes | Serves 4

- 1 cup walnut meat
- 1 can French peas
- 1 tablespoon mayonnaise
- 1 medium lettuce

1. Put the walnut meats in extremely hot water for fifteen minutes.
2. Remove the skins, then cut them into pieces. Set your peas to scald, then set aside.
3. Drain the water from the peas and let it get cold; then mix with the walnuts.
4. Add the mayonnaise dressing and mix thoroughly. Serve on lettuce.

PER SERVING

Calories: 252 | Fat: 2g | Carbohydrates: 11g | Fiber: 4g | Protein: 10g

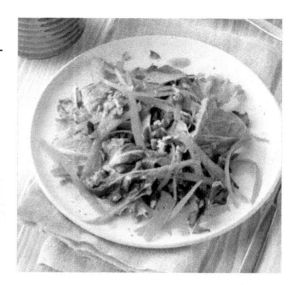

Chapter 10
Desserts

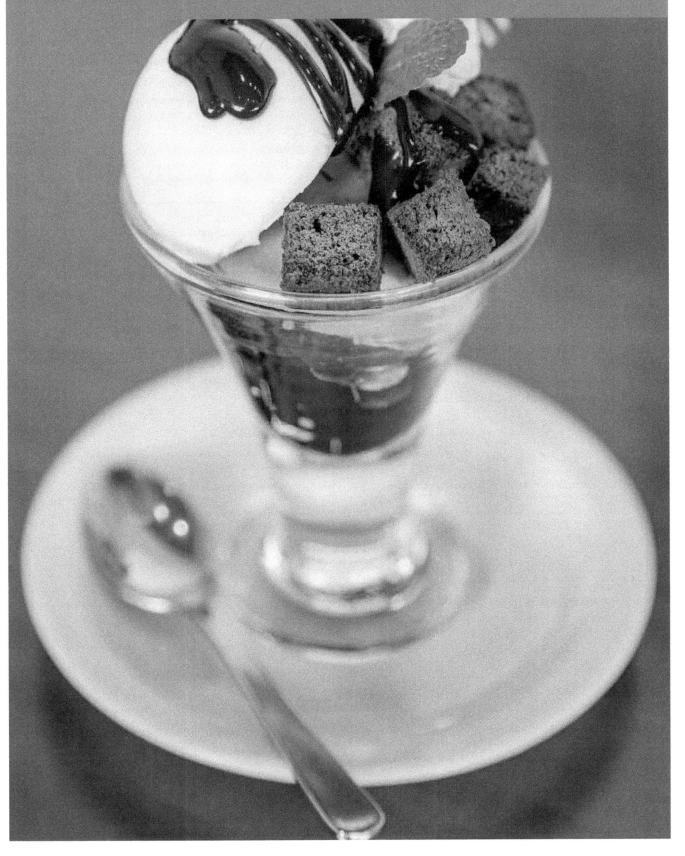

Papaya-Mango Smoothie

Prep time: 5 minutes | Cook time: 0 minutes |Serves 2

- 1 cup mango, diced
- 1 cup papaya chunks
- 1 cup almond or lactose-free milk
- 1 tablespoon honey or maple syrup

1. Blend all ingredients in a blender and then pulse until smooth.
2. Pour into a large glass. Enjoy!

PER SERVING

Calories: 554 | Fat: 32g | Carbohydrates: 14g | Sugar: 8g | Fiber: 2g | Protein: 50g | Sodium: 632 mg

Cantaloupe Smoothie

Prep time: 5 minutes | Cook time: 0 minutes |Serves 2

- 1 cup cantaloupe, diced
- 1/2 cup vanilla yogurt or lactose-free yogurt
- 1/2 cup orange juice
- 1 tablespoon honey or maple syrup
- 2 ice cubes

1. Merge all ingredients in a blender and then pulse until smooth.
2. Pour into a large glass. Enjoy!

PER SERVING

Calories: 179 | Fat: 13g | Carbohydrates: 6g | Sugar: 3g | Fiber: 1g | Protein: 10g | Sodium: 265 mg

Cantaloupe-Mix Smoothie

Prep time: 5-10 minutes | Cook time: 0 minutes |Serves 2

- 1 cup cantaloupe, diced
- 1/2 cup mango, diced
- 1/2 cup almond milk or lactose-free cow milk
- 1/2 cup orange juice
- 2 tablespoons lemon
- 1 tablespoon honey or maple syrup
- 2 ice cubes

1. Merge all ingredients in a blender until smooth.
2. Pour into a large glass. Enjoy!

PER SERVING

Calories: 329 | Fat: 17g | Carbohydrates: 9g | Sugar: 3g | Fiber: 5g | Protein: 37g | Sodium: 430 mg

Applesauce-Avocado Smoothie

Prep time: 5-10 minutes | Cook time: 0 minutes |Serves 1

- 1 cup unsweetened almond or lactose-free milk
- 1/2 avocado
- 1/2 cup applesauce
- 1/4 teaspoon ground cinnamon
- 1/2 cup ice
- 1/2 teaspoon stevia or 1 tablespoon honey for sweetness (optional)

1. Blend all ingredients in a blender. Pulse the mix until smooth.
2. Pour into a large glass. Enjoy!

PER SERVING

Calories: 270 | Fat: 11g | Carbohydrates: 4g | Sugar: 1g | Fiber: 1g | Protein: 39g | Sodium: 664 mg

Pina Colada Smoothie

Prep time: 5-10 minutes | Cook time: 0 minutes |Serves 1

- 1 cup papaya chunks
- 1/2 cup unsweetened almond milk or lactose-free milk
- 1 banana
- 1/2 teaspoon vanilla extract, to taste
- 1 tablespoon honey, maple syrup or 1 teaspoon stevia (optional)

1. Blend all ingredients in a blender and then pulse until smooth and creamy.
2. Pour into a large glass. Enjoy!

PER SERVING

Calories: 329 | Fat: 17g | Carbohydrates: 9g | Sugar: 3g | Fiber: 5g | Protein: 37g | Sodium: 430 mg

Diced Fruits

Prep time: 10 minutes | Cook time: 40 minutes |Serves 6

- 4 peaches, skin removed and thinly sliced
- 1 lb. apple, pitted and skin removed
- 1 teaspoon cinnamon powder
- 1 cup honey or maple syrup
- 1 teaspoon vanilla extract

1. In a large pot, cook the fruits in boiling water over medium heat until softened.
2. In a large bowl, mix well all ingredients (except the fruits).
3. Pour the syrup over fruits and let the compote be thickened.
4. Pour the compote into a jar. Serve hot or cold. Enjoy!

PER SERVING

Calories: 178 | Fat: 4g | Carbohydrates: 7g | Fiber: 2g | Protein: 27g

Avocado Dip

Prep time: 10 minutes | Cook time: 0 minutes | Serves 4

- 6 avocados, peeled
- 1/2 tablespoon extra-virgin olive oil
- 1/4 cup chopped fresh cilantro
- 2 tablespoons fresh lime juice
- 1 teaspoon fresh lemon juice
- 1/2 teaspoon salt

1. In a large bowl, set avocados with a fork.
2. Add extra-virgin olive oil and the other ingredients. Enjoy!

PER SERVING

Calories: 75 | Carbohydrates: 0.1g | Protein: 13.4g | Fat: 1.7g | Sugar: 0g | Sodium: 253 mg

Homemade Hummus

Prep time: 10 minutes | Cook time: 60 minutes | Serves 4

- 1/4 lb. dried chickpeas (soaked in water for a night)
- 11/2 tablespoon tahini
- 1 tablespoon lemon juice
- 2 tablespoons extra-virgin olive oil, divided
- 1/4 teaspoon cumin powder
- 1/2 teaspoon salt
- 1 tablespoon water
- 1 teaspoon baking soda (optional)
- 1 teaspoon paprika powder (optional)

1. First, you need to soak the chickpeas overnight in water, and optionally, add baking soda to the water.
2. Cook your chickpeas in a large pot with water over medium heat for about 1 hour. Check if they are cooked well by crushing one of them with a fork in your hand.
3. When chickpeas are cooked, drain and put them in a blender.
4. Add 1 tablespoon of extra-virgin olive oil, lemon juice, tahini, cumin powder, and salt to the blender. Blend until your hummus gets a soft, creamy texture equally.
5. Drizzle with 1 tablespoon of extra-virgin olive oil or paprika powder (optional).
6. Serve immediately or fridge it.

PER SERVING

Calories: 207 | Fat: 16g | Carbohydrates: 5g | Sugar: 2g | Fiber: 1g | Protein: 12g | Sodium: 366 mg

Tofu

Prep time: 10 minutes | Cook time: 25 minutes | Serves 4

- 1 ½ cup firm tofu, pressed and drained
- 1 avocado, cubed
- 1 tablespoon extra-virgin olive oil
- Salt and pepper to taste

1. Preheat your oven to 400°F.
2. Choose a baking sheet, cover it with parchment paper or spray extra-virgin olive oil. Cut tofu cubes of 1/2 inch and spray extra-virgin olive oil on them.
3. Let it bake for 15 minutes until golden brown and crispy. Flip tofu and cook for another 10 minutes. Remove from the oven. Let it rest for 10 minutes.
4. Cube the avocado on a plate. Add salt and pepper.
5. Mix the tofu with avocado in a bowl. Enjoy!

PER SERVING

Calories: 645 | Fat: 32g | Carbohydrates: 65g | Fiber: 5g | Protein: 26g

Whole-wheat Chocolate Chip Cookies

Prep time: 10 minutes | Cook time: 10 minutes | Serves 48

- 1 cup (225 g) unsalted butter
- 1/4 cup (64 g) peanut butter
- 1 cup (340 g) honey
- 2 eggs
- 1 ½ cup whole-wheat pastry flour
- 1 teaspoon baking soda
- 2 cups (160 g) rolled oats
- 2 cups (350 g) chocolate chips
- 1 cup (110 g) chopped pecans

1. Cream together the first 4 ingredients.
2. Add the next 5 ingredients and mix well.
3. Add enough flour for a stiff dough.
4. Drop by teaspoons on a baking sheet.
5. Bake at 375°F (190°C, gas mark 5) for 10 minutes.

PER SERVING

Calories: 365 | Fat: 7g | Carbohydrates: 67g | Sugar: 16g | Fiber: 18g | Protein: 14g | Sodium: 629 mg | Saturated Fat: 1 g | Cholesterol: 0 g

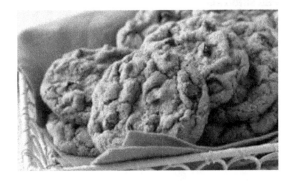

Good for You Chocolate Chip Cookies

Prep time: 10 minutes | Cook time: 10 minutes | Serves 36

- 1/4 cup (55 g) unsalted butter
- 1 cup (150 g) packed brown sugar
- 1/4 cup (85 g) honey
- 1 egg
- 1 teaspoon vanilla extract
- 1/4 cup (60 ml) skim milk
- 1 teaspoon baking soda
- 1/2 teaspoon baking powder
- 1 cup (82 g) granola
- 3/4 cup quick-cooking oats
- 2 cups whole-wheat pastry flour
- 1 cup (175 g) chocolate chips

1. Cream the butter and brown sugar.
2. Mix in honey, egg, vanilla, and milk, then baking soda and baking powder.
3. Add granola, oats, and flour. Mix all ingredients.
4. Stir in chocolate chips.
5. Place on a non-stick baking sheet in teaspoons.
6. Bake at 325°F (170°C, gas mark 3) for 10 minutes.

PER SERVING

Calories: 287 | Fat: 19g | Carbohydrates: 18g | Sugar: 6g | Fiber: 6g | Sodium: 451 g | Saturated Fat: 3 g | Cholesterol: 0 g

Oat and Wheat Cookies

Prep time: 10 minutes | Cook time: 12-15 minutes | Serves 4

- 3/4 cup (165 g) unsalted butter
- 1/2 cup (130 g) peanut butter
- 1 cup (150 g) brown sugar
- 1 ¼ cup (150 g) whole-wheat pastry flour
- 1 teaspoon baking soda
- 1 ¼ cup (100 g) rolled oats

1. Mix all ingredients.
2. Set by rounded teaspoons onto an ungreased baking sheet.
3. Bake at 375°F (190°C, gas mark 5) for 10–12 minutes or until golden brown.
4. Let rest on the baking sheet for 1 minute and then cool on racks.

PER SERVING

Calories: 124 | Fat: 3g | Carbohydrates: 22g | Sugar: 5g | Fiber: 3g | Protein: 2g | Saturated Fat: 0 g | Cholesterol: 0 g

Oatmeal Spice Cookies

Prep time: 10 minutes | Cook time: 30 minutes | Serves 48

- 1 cup (145 g) raisins
- 1 cup (235 ml) water
- 1/2 cup (112 g) unsalted butter, softened
- 1/4 cup (60 ml) vegetable oil
- 1 ½ cup (300 g) sugar
- 2 eggs
- 1 teaspoon vanilla extract
- 2 ½ cups (300 g) whole-wheat pastry flour
- 1/2 teaspoon baking powder
- 1 teaspoon baking soda
- 2 teaspoons cinnamon
- 1/4 teaspoon nutmeg
- 2 cups (160 g) quick-cooking oats
- 1/2 cup (60 g) chopped walnuts

1. Preheat the oven to 350°F (180°C, gas mark 4).
2. Simmer the raisins and water in a saucepan on low until plump, for approximately 20 minutes.
3. Drain the liquid into the measuring cup and add water to make 1/2 cup of liquid.
4. Cream butter, oil, and sugar.
5. Add eggs and vanilla.
6. Stir in the raisin liquid.
7. Sift the flour and spices; add to the sugar mixture.
8. Add oats, nuts, and raisins.
9. Set by rounded teaspoons onto an ungreased baking sheet.
10. Flatten slightly and then bake 8–10 minutes or until slightly brown.

PER SERVING

Calories: 357 | Carbohydrates: 54g | Sugar: 5g | Protein: 14g | Sodium: 768 mg | Cholesterol: 8 g

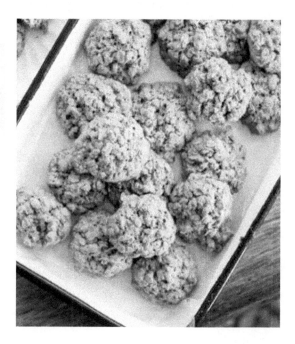

Trail Mix Cookies
Prep time: 10 minutes | **Cook time:** 10 minutes | **Serves 60**

- 3/4 cup (165 g) unsalted butter
- 3/4 cup (150 g) sugar
- 1 egg
- 1 teaspoon vanilla extract
- 2 cups whole-wheat pastry flour
- 1 teaspoon baking soda
- 1 teaspoon cinnamon
- 1/4 teaspoon nutmeg
- 3/4 cup (175 ml) skim milk
- 1 ¾ cup (140 g) quick-cooking oats
- 1 ½ cup (200 g) trail mix

1. Cream the butter and sugar. Add egg and vanilla; beat well. Stir the dry ingredients.
2. Attach them to the mixture alternately with milk, mixing well.
3. Stir in oats and the trail mix. Set by tablespoons on a baking sheet covered with non-stick vegetable oil spray.
4. Bake at 400°F (200°C, gas mark 6) until lightly browned, 8–10 minutes.

PER SERVING
Calories: 413 | Fat: 20g | Carbohydrates: 7g | Sugar: 1g | Fiber: 1g | Protein: 50g | Sodium: 358 mg

White Chocolate Cranberry Cookies
Prep time: 10 minutes | **Cook time:** 10 minutes | **Serves 36**

- 1/2 cup (112 g) shortening
- 1 cup (225 g) brown sugar
- 1 egg
- 1 teaspoon vanilla extract
- 13/4 cups (210 g) whole-wheat pastry flour
- 1 teaspoon baking soda
- 1/4 cup (60 ml) buttermilk
- 1/2 cup (87 g) white chocolate chips
- 1/2 cup (60 g) dried cranberries

1. Beat the shortening until light. Add sugar and beat until fluffy.
2. Beat in the egg and vanilla.
3. Stir the dry ingredients. Attach them to mixture alternately with buttermilk.
4. Beat until smooth. Stir in chips and cranberries.
5. Drop about 2 inches (5 cm) apart on a baking sheet coated with non-stick vegetable oil spray.
6. Bake at 375°F (190°C, gas mark 5) for 8–10 minutes, until lightly browned.

PER SERVING
Calories: 361 | Fat: 10g | Fiber: 14g | Sodium: 139 mg | Saturated Fat: 2 g | Cholesterol: 0 g

Oatmeal Sunflower Bread
Prep time: 10 minutes | **Cook time:** 20 minutes | **Serves 12**

- 1 cup (235 ml) water
- 1/4 cup (85 g) honey
- 2 tablespoons (28 g) unsalted butter
- 3 cups (411 g) bread flour
- 1/2 cup (40 g) quick-cooking oats
- 2 tablespoons non-fat dry milk powder
- 2 teaspoons yeast
- 1 tablespoon vital wheat gluten
- 1/2 cup (72 g) unsalted shelled sunflower seeds

1. Set all ingredients except the sunflower seeds in a bread machine in order specified by the manufacturer.
2. Process on a large white loaf cycle.
3. Add the sunflower seeds at the beep or 5 minutes before the end of kneading.

PER SERVING
Calories: 599 | Fat: 19g | Carbohydrates: 9g | Sugar: 4g | Fiber: 2g | Protein: 97g | Sodium: 520 mg

Maple Oatmeal Bread
Prep time: 10 minutes | **Cook time:** 20 minutes | **Serves 12**

- 1 ¾ teaspoon yeast
- 1 cup (157 ml) warm water
- 2 ½ cups (342 g) bread flour
- 1/2 cup flour
- 1 cup (27 g) rolled oats
- 1 cup (80 ml) maple syrup
- 1/4 cup (17 g) non-fat dry milk
- 2 tablespoons (28 g) unsalted butter, room temperature

1. Add all ingredients to the bread machine in the order specified by the manufacturer.
2. Process on a sweet bread or whole-wheat cycle.

PER SERVING
Calories: 238 | Carbohydrates: 27g | Sugar: 12g | Fiber: 6g | Protein: 21g | Saturated Fat: 2 g | Cholesterol: 39 g

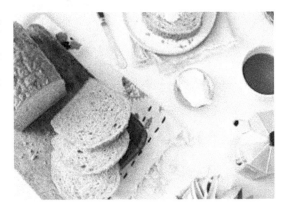

German Dark Bread

Prep time: 10 minutes | Cook time: 20 minutes | Serves 12

- 1 cup (235 ml) water
- 1/4 cup (85 g) molasses
- 1 tablespoon unsalted butter
- 2 cups (274 g) bread flour
- 1 ¼ cup (160 g) rye flour
- 2 tablespoons cocoa powder
- 1 ½ teaspoon yeast
- 1 tablespoon vital wheat gluten

1. Set all ingredients in the bread machine in order specified by the manufacturer.
2. Process on a whole-wheat cycle.

PER SERVING
Calories: 287 | Fat: 9g | Carbohydrates: 18g | Fiber: 6g | Sodium: 451 mg | Saturated Fat: 3 g | Cholesterol: 0 g

Onion and Garlic Wheat Bread

Prep time: 10 minutes | Cook time: 20 minutes | Serves 12

- 1/2 cup (80 g) finely chopped onion
- 1/2 teaspoon finely chopped garlic
- 1 tablespoon sugar
- 1/2 cup whole-wheat flour
- 2 ½ cups (342 g) bread flour
- 1 ½ tablespoon non-fat dry milk
- 1 ½ teaspoon yeast
- 3/4 cup (175 ml) water
- 1 ½ tablespoon (21 g) unsalted butter

1. Set all ingredients in the bread machine in order specified by the manufacturer.
2. Process on a white bread cycle.

PER SERVING
Calories: 329 | Fat: 17g | Carbohydrates: 9g | Sugar: 3g | Fiber: 5g | Protein: 37g

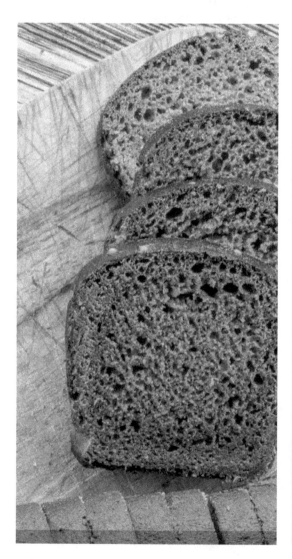

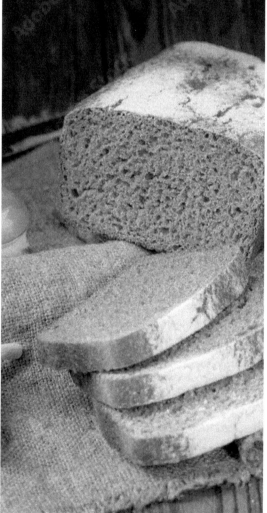

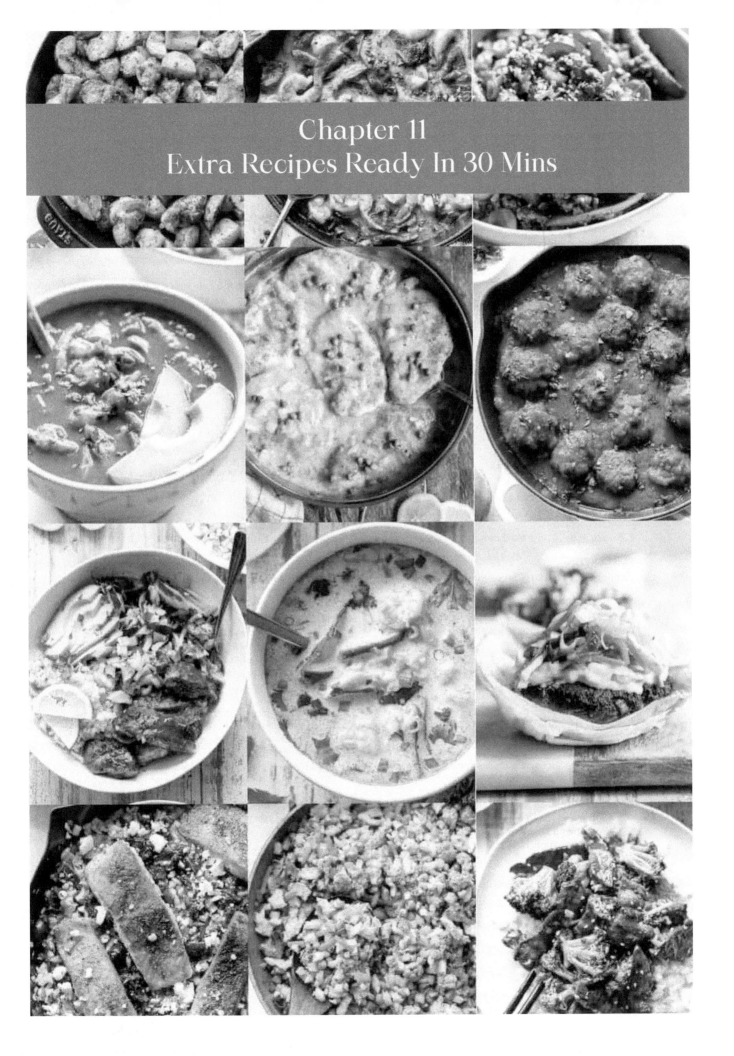
Chapter 11
Extra Recipes Ready In 30 Mins

Smoothie with Mixed Berries
Prep time: 5 minutes | Cook time: 6 minutes | Serves 2

- ½ cup Dairy-Free Yogurt
- 12 ounces Frozen Mixed Berries
- 1 tbsp Honey

1. Combine the water, spinach, and orange juice in a blender, and blend until smooth.
2. Blend in the peanut butter or almond butter until creamy.
3. Blend in the frozen mango and banana until smooth.
4. Finally, serve and enjoy!

PER SERVING

Calories: 265 | Fat: 1g | Carbohydrates: 64g | Protein: 5g

Fruit Punch
Prep time: 5 minutes | Cook time: 10 minutes | Serves 10

- 4 cups Cranberry Juice
- 3 cups, chilled Ginger Ale
- ¼ cup Lime Juice
- 1½ cups Orange Juice
- 1½ cups Pineapple Juice

1. In a pitcher, combine the lime juice, orange juice, cranberry juice, and pineapple juice and chill for one hour.
2. Stir in the ginger ale thoroughly

PER SERVING

Calories: 37 | Fat: 0.2g | Carbohydrates: 11g | Protein: 2g

Chocolate Pudding
Prep time: 5 minutes | Cook time: 10-15 minutes | Serves 7-8

- ½ cup Baking Cocoa
- ¼ cup Cornstarch
- 2 tbsp Dairy-Free Butter
- 4 cups, almond milk Dairy-Free Milk
- ½ tsp Salt
- 1 cup Sugar
- 2 tsp Vanilla Extract

1. Into the saucepan, combine the salt, cornstarch, cocoa, and sugar. Gradually add dairy-free milk. Bring to a boil for two minutes over medium heat.
2. Take the pan off the heat. Stir in the dairy-free butter and vanilla extract well.
3. Pour the pudding into the serving bowl. Refrigerate until ready to serve!

PER SERVING

Calories: 195 | Fat: 5g | Carbohydrates: 37g | Protein: 7g

Soup with Mushroom
Prep time: 10 minutes | Cook time: 20 minutes | Serves 6

- 6 tbsp All-Purpose Flour
- 28 ounces Chicken Broth
- 2 tbsp Dairy-Free Butter
- ½ lb, sliced Mushrooms
- ¼ cup, chopped Green Onion
- ½ tsp Salt

1. Melt the dairy-free butter in the saucepan over medium-high flame. Sauté the green onion (just the green part) and mushrooms until soft.
2. Toss the mushroom mixture with 14 ounces of chicken broth, salt, and flour, and whisk well. Then, after two minutes, add the remaining 14 ounces of broth and bring to a boil.
3. Reduce the heat to low. Cook for fifteen minutes and stir frequently.
4. Finally, serve and enjoy!

PER SERVING

Calories: 133 | Fat: 9g | Carbohydrates: 11g | Protein: 5g

Soup with Broccoli
Prep time: 5 minutes | Cook time: 25 minutes | Serves 4

- ¼ cup All-Purpose Flour
- ¼ tsp Black Pepper
- 2, peeled and sliced Carrots
- 2 cups Chicken Broth
- 1 tbsp plus ¼ cup Dairy-Free Butter
- 12 ounces, chopped Fresh Broccoli
- 1, chopped, green part only Green Onion
- ½ tsp Mustard

1. Melt one tablespoon of diary-free butter in a Dutch oven over medium heat. Then add the green onion (just the green part) and cook for 2 to 3 minutes, or until translucent.
2. Melt ¼ cup of dairy-free butter in the Dutch oven over medium heat. Cook for two minutes after adding flour.
3. Pour in the chicken broth. Let it simmer for two minutes. Using a whisk, mix the ingredients until no lumps remain. After that, toss in the carrots and broccoli thoroughly.
4. Stir in the salt, pepper, and mustard. Reduce the fire to a minimum. Now, slowly simmer for ten minutes.
5. Now, pour the soup into a blender and reduce it to a puree until smooth. If desired, season with pepper and salt.

PER SERVING

Calories: 209 | Fat: 12.1g | Carbohydrates: 16g | Protein: 11g

Wonton Broth

Prep time: 13 minutes | Cook time: 15 minutes | Serves 4

- four, halved lengthwise and halved Baby Bok Choy
- six cups, low sodium Chicken Broth
- one piece, sliced thinly Fresh Ginger
- one clove, minced Garlic
- 1 ½ cups, sliced Mushrooms
- one tsp Sesame Oil
- one tbsp Soy Sauce
- Twenty Wontons

1. First, bring the chicken stock to a boil in a pot.
2. Using a knife, smash and cut the ginger.
3. Place it in the saucepan and cover it with a lid. Allow for five minutes of cooking time.
4. After that, add the bok choy and simmer for another five minutes.
5. Add mushrooms and wontons and continue to cook for another two to three minutes, or until they are soft and wilted.
6. Stir in the sesame oil and soy sauce well.
7. Strain the broth through a sieve.
8. Finally, serve and enjoy!

PER SERVING

Calories: 135 | Fat: 2g | Carbohydrates: 21.5g | Protein: 11g

Cauliflower Broth

Prep time: 10 minutes | Cook time: 20 minutes | Serves 8

- 3 tbsp All-Purpose Flour
- 3 tbsp Butter
- 1, shredded Carrot
- ¼ cup, chopped Celery
- 1 cup, shredded Cheddar Cheese
- 2 tsp Chicken Bouillon
- ½ to one tsp, optional Hot Hepper Sauce
- 1/8 tsp Pepper
- ¾ tsp Salt
- 2 ½ cups Water

1. In a Dutch oven, combine the bouillon, water, celery, carrot, and cauliflower and bring to a boil. Lower the heat. Cover the Dutch oven with a lid.
2. Simmer for 11 to 15 minutes, or until vegetables are soft.
3. Add butter into the saucepan melt it over medium flame.
4. Stir in the pepper, salt, and flour thoroughly. Then, over medium heat, add the milk and bring to a boil. Cook for two minutes, or until the sauce has thickened.
5. Turn down the heat. Stir in the cheese and spicy pepper sauce well. Add cauliflower mixture and mix well.
6. Strain the broth into the basin using a fine mesh strainer.
7. Finally, serve and enjoy!

PER SERVING

Calories: 157 | Fat: 9g | Carbohydrates: 10.7g | Protein: 8g

Ginger Juice

Prep time: 5 minutes | Cook time: 20-25 minutes | Serves 7

- 4 ounces Fresh Ginger Root
- 14-16 leaves Fresh Mint
- 2, juiced Lemons
- 1 cup Sugar or Honey
- 6 to seven cups Water

1. Peel ginger with a knife and discard skin.
2. Break mint into the bowl with a pestle and keep it aside.
3. Chop the ginger into chunks and put it in the blender.
4. Add seven cups of water into the pot and boil it.
5. Add ginger into a blender and then add one cup water and blend until thick.
6. Add ginger paste, mint, and boiled water into the bowl.
7. Strain the contents into the basin using a sieve. Solid parts should be discarded.
8. Toss in the sugar and lemon juice, and serve.

PER SERVING

Calories: 133 | Fat: 1g | Carbohydrates: 33g | Protein: 2g

Lemon Tea

Prep time: 4 minutes | Cook time: 5 minutes | Serves 2

- 2 tsp Back Tea
- 2 tsp Honey
- 1 tbsp Lemon Juice
- 2 cups Water

1. Add water into the pan and heat it.
2. Let simmer it and then add tea leaves. Let steep for one minute.
3. Pass tea through a strainer into the serving cups.
4. Stir in the honey and lemon juice thoroughly
5. Finally, serve and enjoy!

PER SERVING

Calories: 22 | Fat: 1g | Carbohydrates: 5g | Protein: 2g

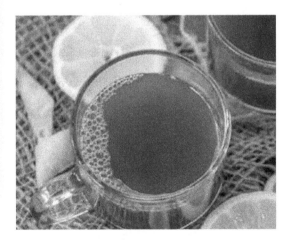

Soup with Red Lentils and Coconut
Prep time: 10 minutes | Cook time: 20 minutes | Serves 6

- 1 cup, chopped Carrot
- ¼ tsp Cayenne Pepper
- 1 cup, full-fat Coconut Milk
- 2 tbsp Olive oil
- 1 cup Fresh Cilantro Leaves
- 3 tbsp Fresh Lime Juice
- 1 cup, chopped, green part only Green Onion
- 1/3 cup Red Curry Paste
- 1 cup Red Lentils
- to taste Salt
- 3 tbsp Tomato Paste
- 4 cups Water

1. Add oil into the Dutch oven and place it over medium flame.
2. Then, add the green onion and carrot and cook for 5 minutes. Add cayenne pepper, curry paste, and tomato paste and cook for one minute until fragrant.
3. Lower the heat to medium-low. Cover the pan with a lid. Let cook for 20 minutes until softened.
4. Remove from the flame. Stir in the lime juice and coconut milk thoroughly.
5. Sprinkle with salt if needed. Garnish with fresh cilantro leaves.

PER SERVING
Calories: 265 | Fat: 13g | Carbohydrates: 27g | Protein: 11g

Soup with Asparagus
Prep time: 5-6 minutes | Cook time: 20 minutes | Serves 6

- 2lbs, cut into 1-inch pieces Asparagus,
- 4 cups Chicken Broth
- 2 tbsp Dairy-Free Butter
- ½ cup Dairy-Free Heavy Cream
- 2 tbsp Flour
- 1, chopped, green part only Green Onion,
- 1 tbsp Olive Oil
- 1 tsp Pepper
- 1 tsp Salt

1. Add olive oil into the pot and place it over medium-high flame.
2. Add green onion and sauté for three to five minutes until tender.
3. Add flour and dairy-free butter and cook until golden brown.
4. Add asparagus and chicken broth and bring to a boil, about seven to ten minutes.
5. Puree the soup in an immersion blender until smooth.
6. Add dairy-free heavy cream and sprinkle with pepper and salt.

PER SERVING
Calories: 179 | Fat: 13g | Carbohydrates: 11g | Protein: 6g

Mashed Sweet Potatoes
Prep time: 9 minutes | Cook time: 20 minutes | Serves 10

- 1 tbsp Brown Sugar
- ¼ tsp Cinnamon
- 1/8 tsp Nutmeg
- 3 pounds, peeled and cube Sweet Potatoes

1. Add peeled and cubed sweet potatoes into the pot and cover with water. Bring to a boil until tender. Drain and place back to the pot.
2. Using a potato masher, mash the potatoes.
3. Add maple syrup, cinnamon, nutmeg, dairy-free butter, and brown sugar and combine with a hand mixer. Finally, serve and enjoy!

PER SERVING
Calories: 191 | Fat: 7g | Carbohydrates: 29g | Protein: 2g

Zucchini Soup
Prep time: 9 minutes | Cook time: 15 minutes | Serves 4

- 1 tbsp Fresh Thyme Leaves
- 1, green part only Green Onion
- 1 cup Raw Cashews
- to taste Salt and Pepper
- 3 Thyme Spears
- 3 Zucchini

1. Soak the cashews in the boiling water.
2. Cut the green onion and zucchini into big chunks.
3. Add green onion and zucchini into the pot. Cover with water. Add thyme spears and bring to a boil for fifteen minutes.
4. Pour it into a blender and puree until smooth.
5. Add pepper, salt, cashews, and one tbsp thyme leaves and blend until smooth.

PER SERVING
Calories: 179 | Fat: 7g | Carbohydrates: 26g | Protein: 8g

Ginger and Mushroom Broth
Prep time: 4 minutes | Cook time: 7 minutes | Serves 4

- 2 tbsp, chopped Basil
- 1 tbsp, grated and peeled Ginger
- ½ cup, chopped Green Onions
- 28 ounces, fat-free Low-Sodium Chicken Broth
- 1 tsp, low-sodium Soy Sauce

1. Place the ginger and mushroom in a saucepan and cook for 2 minutes over medium-high heat. After that, add the soy sauce and chicken stock and bring it to a boil.
2. Add onion and basil and heat it.
3. Strain the soup and serve immediately

PER SERVING
Calories: 71 | Carbohydrates: 14.1g | Protein: 5.2g

Ginger Root Tea
Prep time: 4 minutes | Cook time: 20 minutes | Serves 2

- 2 tbsp Fresh Ginger Root
- 1 tbsp, optional Fresh Lime Juice
- 1 to 2 tbsp Honey
- 4 cups Water

1. Peel the ginger, then cut it into pieces.
2. Place the sliced ginger in the pot with the water and bring to a boil for ten minutes.
3. Allow to boil for 20 minutes. When you're finished, turn off the flame.
4. Strain the tea and then add the lime juice and honey. Finally, serve and enjoy.

PER SERVING

Calories: 39 | Fat: 0g | Carbohydrates: 11.2g | Protein: 0g

Gummies Made with Strawberries
Prep time: 9 minutes | Cook time: 6 minutes

- 1 cup Strawberry Puree
- 2-3 tbsp Honey
- ½ tsp Vanilla Extract
- 1/3 cup Water
- 4 tbsp, un-flavored, grass-fed Gelatin Powder

1. In a medium-sized saucepan, combine the vanilla essence, honey, and strawberry puree and cook for two to four minutes over medium-low heat.
2. Fill the bowl halfway with water, then add the gelatin powder. Stir everything together thoroughly
3. Turn off the flame and add gelatin mixture into the saucepan and whisk it well.
4. Place mixture into the molds and put it into the refrigerator.

PER SERVING

Calories: 6.8 | Fat: 0.1g | Carbohydrates: 1.1g | Protein: 0.6g

Smoothie with Creamy Cherries
Prep time: 5 minutes | Cook time: 4 minutes | Serves 4

- ¼, ripe Avocado
- 1 Cherry
- 1 tbsp Coconut Crème
- 100ml Dark Cherry Juice
- 1 tsp Lecithin Granules
- 1 tsp, hulled Tahini
- 150ml Unsweetened Oat Milk

1. Add all ingredients into the blender. Blend until smooth.
2. Fill the glass halfway with smoothie.

PER SERVING

Calories: 269 | Fat: 9g | Carbohydrates: 59g | Protein: 2g

Lemon Baked Eggs
Prep time: 6 minutes | Cook time: 9 minutes | Serves 1

- 2 slices, low-fat Cheddar Cheese
- 1 Crusty White Roll
- 2g Eggs
- 1 tsp, julienned Lemon
- 2 tbsp, chopped Parsley
- to taste Salt

1. Initially preheat the oven to 180 degrees C.
2. Spray the dish with olive oil.
3. Cut the cheddar cheese into three strips using a sharp knife.
4. Use cheese to line the dishes edges. In the centre of the eggs, crack them.
5. Place julienned lemon over the egg and sprinkle with fresh parsley
6. Place dish into the oven and cook for 9 to 11 minutes. Next serve with crusty white bread rolls.

PER SERVING

Calories: 232 | Carbohydrates: 0.5g | Fat: 15.8g | Protein: 23.3g | Fiber: 3g

Pancakes with Banana
Prep time: 10 minutes | Cook time: 8 minutes | Serves 4

- 1 tbsp Baking Powder
- 2, peeled, sliced Banana
- 2 tsp Cinnamon Powder
- 400ml Dairy-Free Milk
- 349g Firm Silken Tofu
- 250g, gluten-free Flour
- 4 tbsp Grapeseed Oil
- Maple Syrup
- 4 tbsp. Smooth Peanut Butter
- 4 tbsp Sugar
- 1 tbsp Vanilla Extract

1. In a blender, combine the tofu, vanilla, cinnamon, and half of the diary-free milk and blend until smooth.
2. Stir in the remaining diary-free milk.
3. In a separate basin, combine the baking powder and flour. Create a hole in the center of the dry mixture and pour in the wet mixture, blending until smooth.
4. Place the pan over medium heat and add 2 tsp of oil.
5. Pour in the batter and cook for 2 minutes.
6. Flip and cook for another 2 minutes.
7. Spread the pancakes with peanut butter.
8. Finish with sliced bananas as a garnish. Drizzle maple syrup over top.

PER SERVING

Calories: 191 | Carbohydrates: 29.3g | Fat: 6.1g | Protein: 6g | Fiber: 3g

Deviled Egg

Prep time: 5 minutes | Cook time: 10 minutes | Serves 6

- 6 Eggs
- 1 pinch Mustard Powder
- 1 pinch Paprika
- to taste Salt and Pepper
- 1 pinch Turmeric Powder
- 1 packet Water Cracker
- 3 tbsp Whole Egg Mayonnaise

1. Add eggs into the saucepan and cover with water. Place it over medium flame. Bring to a boil. When boiled, cook the eggs for four and a half minutes.
2. Take the pan off the heat. Place the eggs in cold water for one minute.
3. Finally, peel them and cut them in half lengthwise.
4. Remove the yolks from the egg white and add them into the bowl. Let mash with pepper, mustard, mayonnaise, salt and turmeric.
5. Slice a little piece of the rounded bottom of the egg white halves. Place onto the cracker or plate. Place yolk mixture into the white egg halves. Sprinkle with paprika.

PER SERVING

Calories: 121.5 | Carbohydrates: 0.8g | Fat: 10.1g | Protein: 6.1g | Fiber: 2.9g

Muesli Muffins with Pears

Prep time: 6 minutes | Cook time: 20 minutes | Serves 10

- ½ cup Brown Sugar
- 50g, melted Butter
- 1 Egg
- 1 cup Milk
- 150g Muesli
- 2, thinly sliced Pears
- 75g Walnuts
- 200g Wholemeal Self-Rising Flour

1. Initially preheat the oven to 180 degrees C.
2. In a mixing dish, combine the walnuts, pears, sugar, flour, and muesli.
3. In the center of the mixture, make a well.
4. Stir together the butter, milk, and egg in the well.
5. Now spoon the mixture into the muffin tins that have been buttered.
6. Bake for 18 to 20 minutes, sprinkled with muesli.

PER SERVING

Calories: 371 | Carbohydrates: 46g | Fat: 17.9g | Protein: 8g | Fiber: 5g

Shakshuka

Prep time: 10 minutes | Cook time: 15 minutes | Serves 2

- 100g Red Pepper, drained, chopped
- 800g, diced and cooked Tomatoes
- 2 tbsp Tomato Paste
- ½, minced, green part only Green Onion
- 1 ½ tsp Paprika
- 1 tsp Cumin
- ¼ tsp Stevia Powder
- to taste Salt and Pepper
- Olive Oil Spray
- 6 Eggs
- 1 tbsp, chopped Parsley

1. Place a pot over medium flame. Sprinkle with olive oil. Add green onion and cook until translucent.
2. Then, add tomato paste, red pepper, and tomatoes and combine them well. After that, add the stevia and spices to the sauce.
3. Sprinkle with pepper and lower the heat. Over the sauce, crack eggs.
4. Cover the saucepan and cook for 15 minutes on low heat. Finish by garnishing with fresh parsley leaves.

PER SERVING

Calories: 142 | Carbohydrates: 18g | Fat: 10g | Protein: 9g | Fiber: 4g

Salmon Fritter

Prep time: 10 minutes | Cook time: 10-12 minutes | Serves 4

- 400g Cooked White Rice
- 1 Egg
- ½ cup Oats
- 2 tbsp Olive Oil
- 50g Tomato Paste
- 350g, drained Tuna or Salmon
- ¼ cup Wholemeal Flour

1. Initially preheat the oven to 100 degrees C
2. Then, in a bowl, combine the salmon, rice and oats. Make a well in the center and pour in the beaten egg and tomato paste, blending until smooth.
3. Stir in the white flour, then form the mixture into eight patties.
4. Transfer to a baking tray and then bake for 5 minutes.
5. Flip and cook for another five minutes.
6. Toss with tomato sauce and serve.

PER SERVING

Calories: 301 | Carbohydrates: 23.1g | Fat: 9g | Protein: 29g | Fiber: 4g

Vanilla Almond Hot Chocolate

Prep time: 10 minutes | Serves 2

- 600ml Vanilla Almond Milk
- 30g Full Fat Coconut Cream
- 60g Dark Chocolate
- 1 tsp Cocoa
- to taste Stevia

1. Place the pan over medium heat and add the vanilla almond milk.
2. Heat the mixture with the stevia, cocoa powder, and chopped chocolate.
3. Finish with coconut cream and a sprinkling of chocolate shavings.

PER SERVING

Calories: 195 | Carbohydrates: 31g | Fat: 3.8g | Protein: 8.2g | Fiber: 1.2g

Frittata with Spinach

Prep time: 5 minutes | Cook time: 25 minutes | Serves 4

- 1 tbsp Coconut Oil
- 8 Eggs
- 1 cup Egg Whites
- 3 tbsp Milk
- 1, peeled and sliced into thin rings Shallot
- 1 cup, thinly sliced into rings Baby Bell Peppers
- 5 ounces, chopped Fresh Spinach
- 3 ounces, crumbled Feta Cheese
- to taste Salt and Pepper

1. Initially preheat the oven to 200 degrees C.
2. In a large mixing basin, whisk together the salt, milk, egg whites, and egg. Set it aside for now.
3. Preheat the pan over a medium-high heat. After that, pour in the coconut oil into the pan. Add sliced peppers and sliced shallot and sprinkle with pepper and salt. Let cook it for five minutes. Add chopped spinach and stir well.
4. Pour the egg mixture into the pan after whisking it. Sprinkle with the feta cheese.
5. Put it in the oven for ten to twelve minutes to cook. Set aside to cool. Finally, serve and enjoy!

PER SERVING

Calories: 241 | Carbohydrates: 7g | Protein: 23g | Fat: 11g

Smoothie with Banana

Prep time: 5 minutes | Cook time: 5-6 minutes | Serves 1

- 1 cup, sliced Banana
- ¼ cup Greek Yogurt
- ¼ cup Milk
- ¼ tsp Vanilla Extract

1. In a blender, combine all ingredients. Blend until smooth.
2. If necessary, add extra milk.
3. Finally, serve and enjoy!

PER SERVING

Calories: 201 | Carbohydrates: 38g | Protein: 11g | Fat: 2.9g

Muffins with Banana

Prep time: 5 minutes | Cook time: 25 minutes | Serves 10

- 1 ½ cups All-Purpose Flour
- 1 tsp Baking Powder
- 1 tsp Baking Soda
- 3, mashed Bananas
- 1/3 cup, melted Butter
- 1 Egg
- ½ tsp Salt
- ¾ cup Sugar

1. Initially preheat the oven to 180 degrees C.
2. Spray the muffin tins with nonstick cooking spray.
3. Strain the salt, baking powder, baking soda, and flour and keep it aside.
4. In a mixing dish, combine the melted butter, egg, sugar, and bananas.
5. Add flour mixture in it and combine it well.
6. Place mixture into the muffin pans. Bake it for 10/15 minutes.

PER SERVING

Calories: 184 | Carbohydrates: 32.1g | Protein: 2.9g | Fat: 5.7g

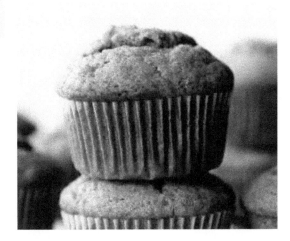

Omelet with Mushrooms

Prep time: 12 minutes | Cook time: 15 minutes | Serves 2

- 1 tbsp, shredded, low-fat Cheddar Cheese
- 1 Egg
- 3 Egg Whites
- ½ cup, sliced Fresh Mushrooms
- 1 cup, torn Fresh Spinach
- ½ cup, diced Fresh Tomato
- 1/8 tsp Garlic Powder
- ¼ cup, diced Green Onion
- 1/8 tsp Ground Black Pepper
- 1/8 tsp Ground Nutmeg
- ½ tsp Olive Oil
- 1 tbsp, grated Parmesan Cheese
- 2 tbsp, chopped Red Bell Pepper
- ¼ tsp Salt

1. First of all, in a mixing dish, whisk together the egg whites and the egg. Then, add pepper, nutmeg, garlic powder, salt, and cheddar cheese and combine it well.
2. Place the skillet over medium heat and add the oil. Add bell pepper, green onion, and mushrooms and cook for five minutes, until tender. Add spinach to the skillet. Cook until wilted.
3. Cook for 12 minutes after adding the egg mixture and sliced tomato.
4. Cut into the wedges. Serve and enjoy!

PER SERVING

Calories: 113 | Carbohydrates: 5.5g | Protein: 12.9g | Fat: 4.9g

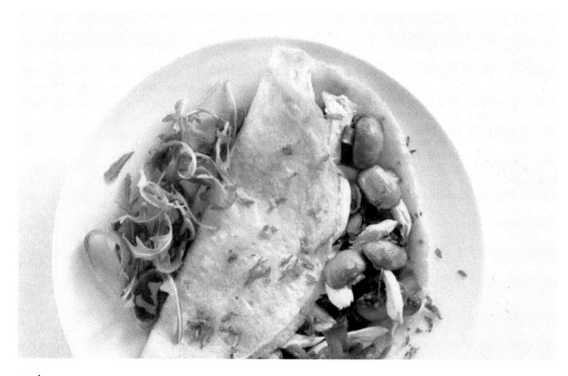

Appendix 1 Measurement Conversion Chart

Volume Equivalents (Dry)	
US STANDARD	**METRIC (APPROXIMATE)**
1/8 teaspoon	0.5 mL
1/4 teaspoon	1 mL
1/2 teaspoon	2 mL
3/4 teaspoon	4 mL
1 teaspoon	5 mL
1 tablespoon	15 mL
1/4 cup	59 mL
1/2 cup	118 mL
3/4 cup	177 mL
1 cup	235 mL
2 cups	475 mL
3 cups	700 mL
4 cups	1 L

Volume Equivalents (Liquid)		
US STANDARD	**US STANDARD (OUNCES)**	**METRIC (APPROXIMATE)**
2 tablespoons	1 fl.oz.	30 mL
1/4 cup	2 fl.oz.	60 mL
1/2 cup	4 fl.oz.	120 mL
1 cup	8 fl.oz.	240 mL
1 1/2 cup	12 fl.oz.	355 mL
2 cups or 1 pint	16 fl.oz.	475 mL
4 cups or 1 quart	32 fl.oz.	1 L
1 gallon	128 fl.oz.	4 L

Temperatures Equivalents	
FAHRENHEIT(F)	**CELSIUS(C) APPROXIMATE)**
225 °F	107 °C
250 °F	120 ° °C
275 °F	135 °C
300 °F	150 °C
325 °F	160 °C
350 °F	180 °C
375 °F	190 °C
400 °F	205 °C
425 °F	220 °C
450 °F	235 °C
475 °F	245 °C
500 °F	260 °C

Weight Equivalents	
US STANDARD	**METRIC (APPROXIMATE)**
1 ounce	28 g
2 ounces	57 g
5 ounces	142 g
10 ounces	284 g
15 ounces	425 g
16 ounces (1 pound)	455 g
1.5 pounds	680 g
2 pounds	907 g

Appendix 2 The Dirty Dozen and Clean Fifteen

The Environmental Working Group (EWG) is a nonprofit, nonpartisan organization dedicated to protecting human health and the environment Its mission is to empower people to live healthier lives in a healthier environment. This organization publishes an annual list of the twelve kinds of produce, in sequence, that have the highest amount of pesticide residue-the Dirty Dozen-as well as a list of the fifteen kinds of produce that have the least amount of pesticide residue-the Clean Fifteen.

THE DIRTY DOZEN	
The 2016 Dirty Dozen includes the following produce. These are considered among the year's most important produce to buy organic:	
Strawberries	Spinach
Apples	Tomatoes
Nectarines	Bell peppers
Peaches	Cherry tomatoes
Celery	Cucumbers
Grapes	Kale/collard greens
Cherries	Hot peppers
The Dirty Dozen list contains two additional items kale/collard greens and hot peppers-because they tend to contain trace levels of highly hazardous pesticides.	

THE CLEAN FIFTEEN	
The least critical to buy organically are the Clean Fifteen list. The following are on the 2016 list:	
Avocados	Papayas
Corn	Kiw
Pineapples	Eggplant
Cabbage	Honeydew
Sweet peas	Grapefruit
Onions	Cantaloupe
Asparagus	Cauliflower
Mangos	
Some of the sweet corn sold in the United States are made from genetically engineered (GE) seedstock. Buy organic varieties of these crops to avoid GE produce.	

Appendix 3 Index

A
abalone 3, 44
all-purpose flour 23, 29, 30, 45, 54, 55, 62, 76, 77, 79, 84, 89
all-purpose white flour 88
almonds 80
Anaheim chile 61, 62
apple 12, 17, 20, 24, 27, 39, 41, 42, 47, 61, 67
apple cider vinegar 91
apple juice 40

B
baby back ribs 68, 73
baking powder 79, 80, 84, 88, 89
baking soda 76, 88
bamboo shoots 44
banana 89
barbecued beef 87

C
cabbage 1, 7, 14, 15, 16, 17, 19, 20, 24, 29, 35, 36, 38, 52, 61, 63, 70, 89
cake flour 79
Canadian bacon 24, 87
cane sugar 22
canola oil 33, 37, 46, 71, 72, 73, 74
capers 40
carrot 14, 15, 16, 22, 23, 24, 27, 29, 33, 37, 41, 42, 45, 49, 51, 52, 54, 56, 57, 58, 59, 61, 62, 64, 78, 83, 89
cashews 88, 89, 91
cayenne pepper 23, 88
chili-garlic oil 90

D
daenjang 6, 12
daikon radish 7, 15, 16, 46, 61, 62
dark brown sugar 25, 42, 44, 57, 80
dashi granules 64
dates 65, 80
doenjang 7, 12, 41, 61, 65, 67
Dongchimi juice 57
dried anchovies 6, 11, 62
dried baby anchovies 83

E
edamame 58
egg 1, 3, 4, 5, 23, 24, 25, 29, 37, 40, 46, 48, 49, 51, 52, 56, 57, 58, 59, 76, 79, 88, 89
eye round steak 40

F
fermented bean paste 64
fish cakes 45, 52
fish sauce 5, 7, 12, 14, 15, 16, 17, 30, 31, 35, 36, 38, 48, 49, 70
flanken-style short ribs 71

G
garlic 6, 7, 9, 11, 12, 14, 15, 16, 17, 18, 19, 20, 23, 24, 25, 27, 28, 30, 31, 32, 33, 35, 36, 37, 38, 39, 40, 41, 42, 44, 45, 46, 47, 49, 51, 52, 53, 54, 55, 56, 57, 58, 61, 62, 63, 64, 65, 67, 68, 69, 70, 71, 72, 73, 83, 84, 85, 88, 89, 90
garlic paste 64
garlic powder 38, 39, 67, 88

H
half-and-half 76
halibut 47
heavy cream 81
heavy whipping cream 76
herbs 37, 71, 72, 73
hoisin sauce 31
Holland chile 45, 46, 47
honey 11, 12, 27, 30, 31, 33, 36, 38, 41, 51, 52, 62, 70, 73, 78, 83
honey powder 52, 62, 69, 76
hot chili oil 67
hot sauce 24, 38
hot sauce glaze 84

I
instant coffee 35, 41
instant dry yeast 76, 77
instant yeast 79

J
jackfruit in brine 25
jalapeño 12, 15, 33, 41, 45, 58
jalapeño chile 15
jalapeno pepper 65
Japanese rice 24
jjolmyeon noodles 56
juice from kimchi 23
jumbo shrimp 44

K
kale 57, 78
ketchup 31, 39, 45
Ketchup 45
Kewpie mayonnaise 22, 24
Korean rice 67, 68, 69, 84, 85
Korean salted shrimp 17, 18, 20
Korean squash 61
Korean udon noodles 55

kosher salt 12, 15, 16, 17, 22, 24, 25, 29, 35, 38, 40, 44, 45, 46, 47, 53, 55, 57, 59, 61, 62, 63, 64, 70, 71, 72, 73, 74, 76, 77, 84

L

lamb ribs 38
large raw shrimp 44
lean ground beef 39, 40, 65
leek 17, 18, 49
lemon 23, 44, 46, 51, 52, 69, 78, 81
lemon juice 23, 44, 46, 56, 88, 91
lemon-lime soda 51
lemon wedge 44, 52
lettuce leaves 5, 23, 28
lettuces 37, 71, 72, 73

M

makgeolli 76
maple syrup 16, 17, 22, 77, 78
masago 52
master anchovy stock 55, 57, 59
master kimchi base 63
mayonnaise 24, 45, 48, 83, 87
milk powder 76

N

Nabak Kimchi 57
naeng myeon noodles 57
napa cabbage 7, 14, 15, 16, 17, 35, 41, 63, 64, 70
napa cabbage kimchee 64
Napa Cabbage Kimchi 14, 51, 67, 68, 76, 87
neutral oil 77
nutritional yeast 89, 91

O

olive oil 28, 29, 38, 40, 46, 47, 55, 56, 57, 59, 78, 87, 88, 89, 90
onion 6, 12, 14, 16, 17, 18, 19, 20, 23, 24, 27, 28, 29, 30, 31, 33, 35, 37, 38, 39, 40, 41, 42, 46, 47, 49, 51, 52, 53, 55, 56, 57, 58, 61, 62, 63, 64, 65, 67, 68, 69, 70, 71, 72, 74, 78, 83, 87, 88, 89, 90
onion powder 67, 88

P

Pacific saury 46
panko bread crumbs 29
peanut oil 48
peanuts 37, 79, 83

Q

quinoa 90

R

radish 7, 14, 15, 17, 18, 19, 24, 35, 37, 46, 47, 55, 59
raisins 80
ramen noodles 58

raw sugar 22
red bell pepper 20, 29, 88
red chile 19, 33, 45, 46, 47
red leaf lettuce 23, 28, 67, 68
red lentils 78
red pepper flakes 23, 40, 87, 89
red snapper 47
rice 1, 6, 7, 9, 11, 12, 15, 16, 17, 19, 20, 22, 23, 24, 25, 27, 28, 29, 30, 31, 32, 33, 36, 37, 38, 39, 40, 41, 42, 44, 46, 47, 51, 52, 53, 54, 57, 58, 59, 61, 62, 63, 65, 67, 69, 70, 71, 72, 73, 76, 80, 85

S

saeujeot 12, 35, 41
sake 31, 45, 59, 61, 67
salmon roe 59
salted belt fish steaks 47
salted shrimp 17, 18, 20, 35

T

tamari 32, 49, 67
toasted nori 51
tobiko 52
tofu 5, 6, 7, 24, 25, 29, 61, 63, 64, 65
tomato paste 29, 89
turbinado sugar 30

U

unflavored rice milk 78
unsalted butter 79
unsweetened shredded coconut 77

V

vanilla extract 88
vanilla ice cream 76
vegetable bouillon 90
vegetable broth 89
vegetable oil 22, 23, 24, 30, 31, 36, 39, 45, 46, 48, 52, 53, 54, 55, 58, 61, 62, 63, 67, 68, 69, 70, 76, 83, 84, 85, 88, 89
vegetable stock 51, 53, 65
vinegar 12, 15, 23, 24, 25, 27, 38, 44, 51, 55, 57, 59, 67, 73, 88
vodka 84, 85

W

walnut halves 23
walnuts 23, 67, 76, 80
watercress 59
whelk juice 83

Y

yubu 87
Yubu chobap seasoning package 87

Z

zucchini 41, 51, 55, 56, 61, 64, 65, 88

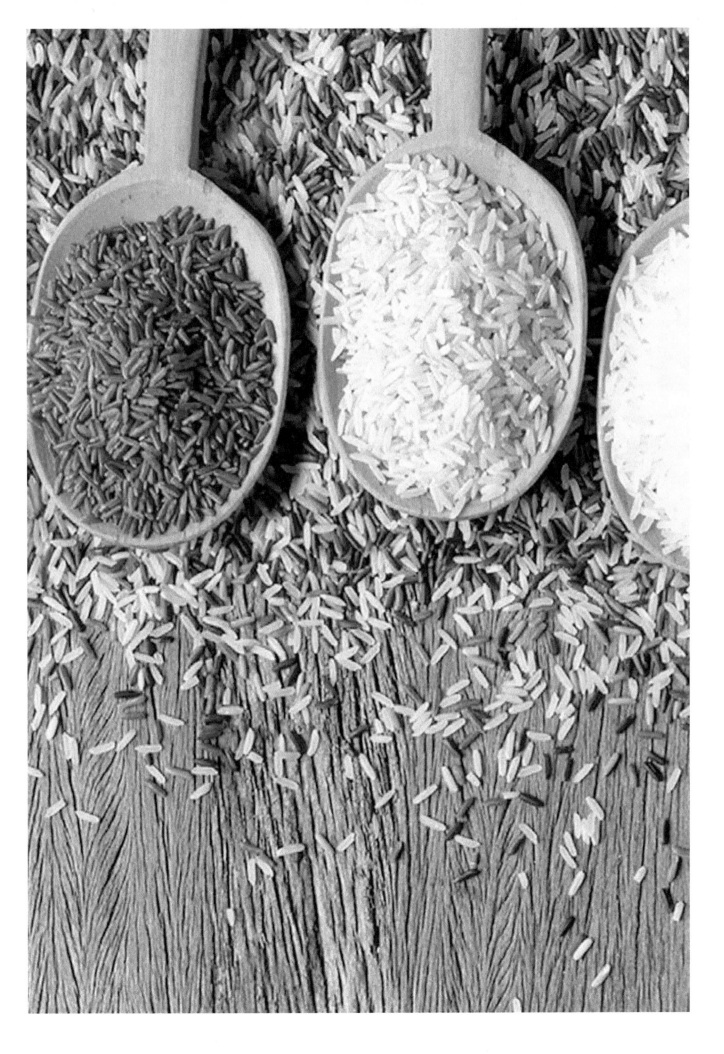

SYLVIA F. OWENS

Printed in the USA
CPSIA information can be obtained
at www.ICGtesting.com
CBHW082142041124
16922CB00010B/209

9 781805 380580